A–Z of Medical Statistics

A COMPANION FOR CRITICAL APPRAISAL

FILOMENA PEREIRA-MAXWELL

MBBS, MSc Clinical Tropical Medicine,
MSc Medical Statistics formerly Lecturer in Medical
Statistics, St Bartholomew's and the Royal London School
of Medicine and Dentistry and member of the
North Thames Research Appraisal Group (NTRAG)

A member of the Hodder Headline Group
LONDON
Co-published in the United States of America by
Oxford University Press Inc., New York

First published in Great Britain in 1998, reprinted 2001 by
Arnold, a member of the Hodder Headline Group,
338 Euston Road, London, NW1 3BH

http://www.arnoldpublishers.com

Co-published in the United States of America by
Oxford University Press Inc.,
198 Madison Avenue, New York, NY10016
Oxford is a registered trademark of Oxford University Press

British Library Cataloguing in Publication Data
A catalogue record for this book is available from the British Library

Library of Congress Cataloging-in-Publication Data
A catalog record for this book is available from the Library of Congress

ISBN 0 340 71940 0 (pb)

4 5 6 7 8 9 10

Publisher: Georgina Bentliff
Project Editor: Catherine Barnes
Production Editor: Wendy Rooke
Production Controller: Sarah Kett

Typeset in 9.5pt Sabon and produced by Gray Publishing, Tunbridge Wells, Kent
Printed and bound in India by Replika Press Pvt Ltd. 100% EOU,
Delhi 110 040

Contents

Foreword

Die Arznei macht kranke, die Mathematik traurige und die Theologie südhafte Leute. (Medicine makes people ill, mathematics makes them sad and theology makes them sinful.) Martin Luther 1483–1546

It seems that medical statistics can also make people feel ill, sad and, if not exactly 'sinful', aware of the short-comings of much medical research. The ideas are complex and can be difficult to understand, yet students and health professionals are under increasing pressure both to pass examinations including statistics and to understand statistical methods used in research.

The medical literature has an increasing emphasis on statistical methods, and with the easy access to sophisticated statistical software the range of techniques used in published papers has burgeoned. Busy medical practitioners cannot be statistical experts but wish to remain up-to-date in their own field. Courses on statistics, however well taught, have a half-life for the technical detail retained in the learners' memories that is at best a few months. Well-taught courses in critical appraisal can teach concepts that may have a much longer retention time. This is not a textbook but, by allowing rapid access to the vocabulary, intends to keep the ideas fresh for those who, having been taught the principles, wish to make regular (possibly infrequent) use of them in practical assessment of the literature.

Dr Pereira-Maxwell is both a physician and a medical statistician whose mother tongue happens not to be English, but who speaks more than one language. Her work in writing this *A–Z* reflects this background. Her careful attention to the problems of understanding the language of medical statistics have been aided by her linguistic heritage. I believe it will be a useful adjunct to the teaching of appraisal skills and to keeping them honed when they are used in medical practice.

Teaching students and practitioners of the health professions who want to learn has been one of the most rewarding experiences of my life. The debt that many of us owe to Professor David Sackett, who has inspired much of the best teaching in this field, is vast. I hope this book helps to keep that type of teaching coruscating without requiring a perfect memory for the words used in papers.

Stephen Evans
Visiting Professor
The London School of Hygiene and Tropical Medicine

Acknowledgements

I wish to acknowledge and express my gratitude to the many authors of medical statistics texts to whom I am indebted. In addition, I would like to thank several people who provided invaluable help with comments, suggestions, ideas, proof-reading and patience. They are Professor Stephen Evans, who suggested this project to me, and whose advice shaped the book's final format; Mike Chambers, former NTRAG academic coordinator; Michele Emerick, former NTRAG administrator; Professor Roger Feldman, Mary Walker, Joe Rosenthal and Rumana Omar, NTRAG tutors; Enid Hennessy, Allan Hackshaw and Joan Morris fellow medical statisticians; Mrs Di Mullineux; Dr Gail Crowe, at the Ambrose King Centre (Royal London Hospital); Professor Graham Dunn, at the University of Manchester (formerly, Institute of Psychiatry, London), for his comments and for allowing me to use his own glossary for multivariate methods; Bill Gould (at StataCorp), Professors Douglas Altman, Beth Dawson-Saunders, David Sackett and Nicholas Wald, for kind permission to use data and reproduce materials; Richard Harris, NTRAG project manager; NTRAG statistics foundation course participants and other NTRAG tutors; my husband Raymond Maxwell, for his support and many cups of tea and coffee; Georgina Bentliff, Catherine Barnes, Wendy Rooke, Sarah Kett and Gavin Armstrong at Arnold, and Robert Gray at Gray Publishing. Last, but not least, my sincere thanks to Dr Richard Morris, whose proof-reading, corrections, amendments and additions have made a major contribution to the contents.

This book has been produced with the help of an NHS (North Thames) R&D grant to the North Thames Research Appraisal Group.

The North Thames Research Appraisal Group

The North Thames Research Appraisal Group (NTRAG) is an education and training consultancy consisting of a mixed group of 35 researchers, academics, clinicians and other health care professionals committed to the promotion of evidence-based healthcare. The means by which they achieve this goal is through the design and delivery of a wide range of critical appraisal skills workshops and related activities for all health care professionals, regardless of professional background or seniority.

The *A–Z of Medical Statistics* was originally commissioned by NTRAG with the aim of providing the participants of its workshops, or anybody else wanting to understand medical research, with an accessible and easy-to-use tool for the appraisal of both its relevance and validity.

NTRAG's overall teaching philosophy supports the view expressed in the UK's National Health Service (NHS) Executive (1996) publication, *Promoting Clinical Effectiveness*: a major policy statement outlining a strategy to help health authorities and trusts promote greater clinical effectiveness. It states that:

> Health Authorities and GP Fund-holders need to take account of the strength of scientific evidence ... about clinical practices and cost-effectiveness when making investments in new and existing services ... Local NHS management should support the use of clinical guidelines, well-targeted post-graduate education and *continuing professional development* [our emphasis] to promote more effective practices. (p 5)

Established in 1993 with funding from the NHS Executive (North Thames), NTRAG's main efforts are devoted to delivering its annual *Improving Clinical Effectiveness* programme of critical appraisal skills workshops. Over the years this programme has grown considerably and now offers over 40 workshops annually covering nine topic areas, all focusing on the critical appraisal of published research.

NTRAG staff and tutors also work with UK trusts, health authorities and other health care organizations to create short-course programmes tailored specifically to local requirements. These *Teaching for Change* activities are generally delivered on-site, enabling educational content to be linked directly to the needs of patients and services. In this way, NTRAG is making an active contribution to the important local change processes that underpin many long-term improvements to health care delivery throughout the UK.

NTRAG is based at the Department of Primary Care and Population Sciences, Royal Free Hospital School of Medicine and University College London, UK.

telephone: +44(0)171-830 2549

e-mail: ntrag@rfhsm.ac.uk

website: http://cebm.jr2.ox.ac.uk/ntrag/ntrag.html

Introduction

Readers of the medical literature are constantly assaulted by the language of statistics and research methodology, while valiantly trying to extract the best clinical evidence available. The *A–Z of Medical Statistics* seeks to provide explanations of terms frequently encountered by readers, in such a way as to clarify their meaning and show the inter-dependency between various important concepts.

The need for a collection of concise explanations of concepts frequently encountered in medical journals became apparent during Critical Appraisal Workshops organized by the North Thames Research Appraisal Group (NTRAG). Concepts such as normality, randomization, standard errors, *P*-values, risk, study design, to name just a few, are rather ubiquitous in the literature. This book has been structured as a dictionary, with substantial cross-referencing between the various entries. It is hoped this will decrease the need for lengthy explanations and unnecessary repetitions, which would defeat the purpose of this companion. In any particular entry, the reader is invited to look up terms highlighted in **bold** for clarification on related concepts, whenever necessary. All terms in **bold** have independent entries.

This book is not intended to replace existing medical statistics textbooks, especially for those wanting to design and carry out research studies. As the reader and appraiser of published medical literature is our primary target, the *A–Z* should make the task less daunting.

Textbooks and papers consulted are listed under references, together with other useful readings. These references mainly include texts which appeal to a non-statistical audience, and may therefore be of value to our intended readership. Formulae for sample size calculation are given in Appendix A. A 'problem-oriented' guide to choosing the appropriate statistical tests, and some worked examples, can be be found in Appendices B and C. Appendix D has some worked examples of the assessment of agreement and reliability of measurements.

A–Z guide

Absolute risk difference (ARD)

or absolute risk reduction (ARR). In comparative studies, the ARD is the difference in **risk** of a particular event, between two groups. As opposed to the **risk ratio**, which only expresses the relative benefits of one treatment compared to another (e.g. *twice as many* patients died on treatment A compared with treatment B), the ARD is dependent on the risk of the event in the **control** group (or baseline risk). The benefits of one treatment compared with the other can therefore be expressed in absolute or net terms. Using the example above, it is possible to state *how many deaths* are prevented by treatment B in comparison with treatment A. The ARR is used to compute the **number needed to treat**, which conveys a similar idea. From Table 1, p 15:

$$\text{ARD} = \text{risk}_2 - \text{risk}_1 = \frac{b}{b+d} - \frac{a}{a+c}$$

where risk_2 is the risk of the event in the control group (baseline risk) and risk_1 is the risk in the treatment or intervention group. The example in Box 1 illustrates these concepts.

BOX 1
ISIS Collaborative Group (1988). Randomized trial of streptokinase, oral aspirin, both, or neither among 17,187 cases of suspected acute myocardial infarction: ISIS-2. *The Lancet* **ii**: 349–359.
In this multicentre clinical trial, over 17 000 patients suspected of having acute myocardial infarction (AMI) were randomized to receive one of the four treatment alternatives mentioned above. This example concentrates on the comparison of all patients receiving aspirin vs all not receiving aspirin (160 mg/day for one month), regardless of any other concomitant treatments. For an explanation of the design used in this study, see **factorial design**. The results are (for vascular mortality at five weeks):

	No. who died (%)	95% CI for difference	P-value	
Aspirin	804/8587 (9.4)			
		1.5 to 3.4%	<0.00001	
No aspirin	1016/8600 (11.8)			
	ARD	**RR**	**RRR**	**NNT**
	0.024 (2.4)	0.80	20%	42 (1/0.024)

This indicates that for each 1000 patients receiving aspirin after suspicion of AMI, as

> opposed to not receiving aspirin, 24 deaths may possibly be prevented. Given the annual mortality rates for ischaemic heart disease (around 100 per 100 000 population in many western countries), the policy of administering aspirin to AMI patients may have considerable impact, despite the modest relative benefit. See explanation of other quantities under the relevant entries. (RR, relative risk; RRR, relative risk reduction; NNT, number needed to treat; CI, confidence interval; *P*-value.)
>
> See also **attributable risk**.

Accuracy

In the context of clinical measurement. Quality of a measurement which is both correct and **precise (1)**. In most instances, precision is less important than correctness. For example, if the true mass of a patient is 67.567 kg, it is preferable to have it measured as 68 kg rather than 70.432 kg. The **reliability** of a measurement method depends on (among other factors) its accuracy.

Adjusted estimates

As opposed to **crude estimates**. In comparative studies, it refers to **estimates** of treatment or **exposure** effect, computed after taking into account other factors which may explain the effects observed. For example, when comparing death **rates** in populations with different age structure, it is necessary to take account of these age differences. A higher crude mortality rate in one area compared with another, could reflect the older population in that area. After age standardization any differences found in mortality rates can be attributed to factors other than age. Methods such as **stratification**, **standardization**, and **multiple regression** are used to make the adjusted comparisons. These methods take **confounding** factors into account (such as age in the above example), producing estimates which are less **biased**. See Box 4, p 14, for an example.

Age-specific rate

Rate or frequency of occurrence of an event in a defined age group.

Analysis of covariance (ANCOVA)

Statistical method for comparing the **means** of a **quantitative variable** between two or more groups (as in **analysis of variance**), whilst taking into account measurements made for one or more other, possibly influential, quantitative variables or covariates. Since these are often **confounders** or baseline measurements, ANCOVA is used to produce **adjusted estimates**. ANCOVA is commonly carried out using **regression** analysis, with **dummy variables** to represent the groups. This is illustrated with the example given in Box 2.

BOX 2

Risk Factors for Osteoporosis Study. (BUPA data set used with kind permission of Professor Nicholas Wald, Wolfson Institute of Preventive Medicine). Information collected includes menopausal status (pre/post), age in years, smoking habits (yes/no) and bone density (study units), among others.

The aim of this study was to identify risk factors for osteoporosis in women, and to quantify the effects of these risk factors on bone density measurements. In this example we look at the effects of menopausal status and age in a random sample of 200 women.

1 The mean age for the premenopausal group is 43.8 years, and for the postmenopausal group 54.5 years.

2 Age is negatively associated with bone density.

3 Without taking age into account, the average bone density difference between the two groups is 5.7 (pre = 42.9, post = 37.2).

4 When age is taken into account, this difference is reduced to 2.6 (the **regression coefficient** for the regression of bone density on menopausal status is now −2.6, i.e. the vertical distance between the two parallel solid lines). Given that the grouping variable has only two levels – pre and post – there is only need for one (no. of groups −1) dummy variable. This variable takes the value of 0 for premenopausal women and 1 for postmenopausal women. The coefficient for this dummy variable is the average difference between the groups. Here, 'pre' is the baseline group.

5 The effect of age is to decrease bone density, on average by 2.9 for each extra 10 years of life (the regression coefficient for age is −0.29).

6 In fact, as can be seen in Figure 1, there is little association between bone density and age in premenopausal women. This suggests an **interaction** between age and menopausal status, i.e. the effect of age is modified by menopausal status (dashed lines).

The relationships in **4**, **5** and **6** are depicted in Figure 1. Other aspects of this dataset are discussed under interaction. Note that bone density is measured on a particular scale not in g/cm^2. There is however a proportional equivalence between the two scales. For full results see LAW et al. (1997).

Analysis of variance (ANOVA)

Significance test for comparing the **means** of a **quantitative variable** between two or more groups. It is an extension of the independent samples **t-test**, used with just two groups. In summary, ANOVA weighs the total **variability** found in an **outcome variable** of interest and divides it into a between-groups component and a within-groups component (each of these further divided by the appropriate number of **degrees of freedom** to produce a mean square). The significance test for differences between groups is based on the comparison of these two components of variability, under the assumption that no differences exist between groups (**null hypothesis**). If

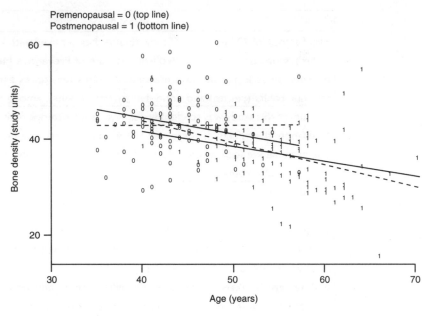

Premenopausal = 0 (top line)
Postmenopausal = 1 (bottom line)

Figure I   Graphical display of an analysis of covariance.

this hypothesis is true, there should be no difference between within and between groups variability, and their ratio is equal to 1. This is known as the **F-test** or variance ratio test. Depending on **study design**, **one-way** or **two-way ANOVA** will be used. Results from ANOVA can be reproduced with some advantages by **regression** methods, using **dummy** or indicator variables to represent the groups.

Area under the curve (AUC)   **Summary measure** used in the context of **repeated measurements analysis,** and **diagnostic testing** using **quantitative** measurements. In the latter context, it is the area below the **ROC** (receiver operating characteristic) **curve** (Figure 16, p 73). Plotting ROC curves for different diagnostic tests enables a comparison of their diagnostic ability to be made: the greater the AUC the better the diagnostic test at correctly identifying individuals with and without a given condition. The area under the curve can thus be interpreted as the probability of correctly identifying the diseased individual and the non-diseased individual, given that one is presented with two subjects randomly selected from a population, where one subject is diseased and the other is not. In repeated measurements analysis the AUC is frequently used instead of the **mean** to convey the idea of response over time, especially when measurements have not been made at equal time intervals, or even when some measurements, but not the last, are missing. Figure 2 shows the diastolic blood pressure (DBP) measurements for two subjects over a period of 2 h after the administration of a hypotensive drug. It can be seen

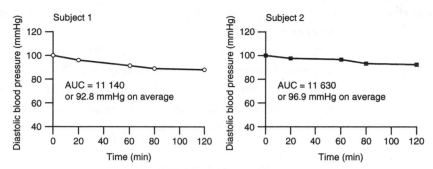

Figure 2 Repeated DBP measurements: AUC.

that subject 2 appears to be less responsive to the drug, and the AUC confirms that on average, over the 120-min period, the DBP for subject 1 was lower by about 4 mmHg. ALTMAN (1991) gives the following formula for calculating the approximate AUC:

$$AUC \approx \frac{1}{2} \sum (y_{i+1} + y_i)(t_{i+1} - t_i)$$

where $\sum$ represents summation, the ys are the measurements and the ts represent time points.

Assumptions

Specific conditions required by **significance tests** and other statistical methods in order to produce valid results. Such methods are usually termed **parametric methods**. Usual assumptions are: **normality** of **distribution** of variables analysed (Figure 10, p 46), **independence** of observations (i.e. coming from different subjects), linear relationship between two variables which are associated, constant variance or **homoscedasticity** (Figure 4, p 8), etc., depending on the statistical method being used. For example, the independent samples **t-test** (for comparing means between two groups) assumes the variable being compared has the same **variance** or **variability** in each of the groups. If this is not the case, the test results may be unreliable.

Attributable risk

Same as **absolute risk difference**. This term is frequently used in the context of epidemiological studies. The attributable risk can also be expressed as a fraction of the **risk** in the **exposed**, the proportional attributable risk or attributable fraction. This is calculated as follows:

$$\text{Proportional attributable risk} = \frac{risk_1 - risk_2}{risk_1} = \frac{RR - 1}{RR}$$

where (from Table 1, p 15) $risk_1$ is the risk in the exposed group and $risk_2$ is the risk in the non-exposed group. The **population attributable risk** measures the impact of a **risk factor** or exposure on a given **population**.

Bar chart   Graphical display of the frequency or relative frequency of the levels of a
categorical variable. It is good practice to separate the bars on the chart,
since the values on the *x*-(horizontal) axis represent 'labels' and have no
numerical meaning (contrast with **histogram**). The bar chart in Figure 3
shows the relative frequency of males and females in a group of first-year
medical students. It can be seen that there are slightly more females than
males, which is the current trend.

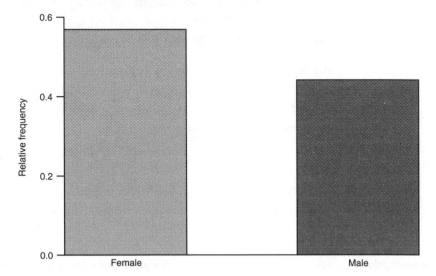

Figure 3 Bar chart.

Bartlett's test   **Significance test** for comparing the **variances** of two or more **populations**.
This test is an extension of the ***F*-test**.

Bayes'   Mathematical equation which gives the conditional probability of an event,
theorem   i.e. the probability that an event will occur *given* that another condition is
also present. This is the basis for the calculation of the probability of disease
given the results of relevant **diagnostic tests**.

Berkson's   Common type of **bias** in **case-control studies,** in particular hospital-based
fallacy   and practice-based studies. It occurs due to differential admission (or
consultation) **rates** between cases and **controls** who have the **risk factor**
being investigated. This leads to positive (and spurious) associations between
exposure and the case-control status with the highest exposure-linked
admission rate. For Berkson's fallacy to occur, the exposure of interest must
itself be an 'admittable' condition. An example would be a case-control study
where cases are patients with stomach cancer and exposure is history of
cirrhosis of the liver. Two scenarios are possible: cases with history of

cirrhosis of the liver are more likely to be admitted (or to consult a doctor) than controls with cirrhosis of the liver, or they are less likely (maybe because of higher mortality). The first scenario may lead to a spurious positive association between disease and exposure, and the second to a negative association (i.e. exposure is protective). See ANDERSEN (1990) and SACKETT (1979) for a full discussion and examples.

Bias

or systematic error. Unlike **random** error, it leads to results which are consistently wrong in one or another direction. Bias can occur in all **study designs** in the form of **selection biases, information biases** and **confounding**. These are broad categories commonly used in the literature. SACKETT (1979) provides a more comprehensive discussion of bias in analytical research. When bias is present in an investigation, the **validity (2)** of its results will be open to question.

Binary variable

Categorical variable which takes only two possible values, for example, yes/no, dead/alive or positive/negative.

Blinding

or masking. In the context of **clinical trials**, whenever participants (single blind trial) or both participants and researchers (double blind trial) are kept unaware of treatments given or received. This avoids the occurrence of observer and respondent biases (**information biases**). In trials comparing an active treatment with no treatment, **placebos** are usually administered to patients in the **control** group to maintain the blinding.

Bonferroni correction

Procedure frequently used in the context of **multiple significance testing**, i.e. when several **significance tests** are carried out simultaneously on the same body of data. Method of keeping the overall probability of wrongly rejecting the **null hypothesis (type I error)** below a specified level, usually 0.05 or 5%. The correction is applied by multiplying each **P-value** obtained by the number of tests performed. If, for example, two groups of patients are compared with respect to three different **outcomes** (say, blood pressure, weight and heart rate) and a *P*-value of 0.04 (**statistically significant** using the conventional cut-off point of 0.05) is obtained for each of these comparisons, then the value for *P* becomes 0.04×3 = 0.12, which is no longer significant. This is a simplified explanation of the method which also takes **sample size** into account. The method tends to give over-corrected *P*-values. *P*-value corrections can also be obtained with **Dunnett's** method.

Bootstrapping	Empirical method of obtaining **confidence intervals (CI)** for **estimates**, which is used when an appropriate mathematical formula does not exist, or when the **assumptions** for using existing formulae are not tenable. This is done by taking a large number of repeated '**samples**' from a single data set (the study sample data), usually using a computer. For example, to obtain a confidence interval for a **mean**, the mean for each 'sample' is calculated. The confidence interval is based on the **distribution** of these 'sample' means, and can be constructed by finding the 2.5th and the 97.5th **percentiles** of this distribution, for a 95% CI.
Box-and-whisker plot	Graphical method for displaying **ordinal variables**. Also useful to describe **quantitative variables** which have a **skewed distribution**. Figure 4 compares the distribution of carboxyhaemoglobin in smokers and non-smokers. It can be seen that this is higher, on average, for smokers, and that for the latter, the measurement has greater **variability**. The 'box' represents the central 50% of the data, and is further divided in two halves by the **median**. The upper and lower boundaries of the 'box' represent the upper and lower **quartiles** (**interquartile range**). The 'whiskers' usually represent the minimum and maximum values of the variable in question. **Outlying** observations can be marked outside the 'whiskers'.

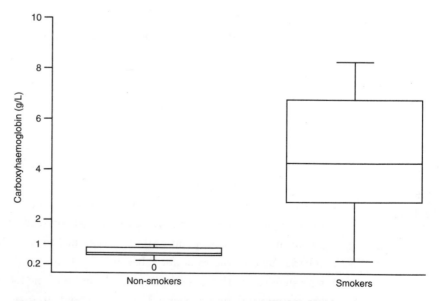

Figure 4 Box-and-whisker plot: unequal variability (BUPA data set used with kind permission of Professor Nicholas Wald, Wolfson Institute of Preventive Medicine, London).

Carry-over effect

In the context of **crossover trials**, occurs when the treatment given in a period of the trial continues to exert an effect into the next period. It is important to evaluate to what extent the effects observed in this period (and attributed to the treatment given here) are a result of or a response to the treatment given in the previous period. Carry-over effects may give rise to **treatment-period interactions**. Appropriate **wash-out periods** between treatments are important in preventing carry-over effects.

Case-control study

Analytical **observational study** which aims to investigate the relationship between an **exposure** or **risk factor** and one or more **outcomes**. This is done by selecting a group of subjects known to have the outcome or disease of interest – known as 'cases', and comparing them with a group of subjects known not to have the disease in question – the **controls** (commonly selected through some form of **matching**). All subjects are then assessed with respect to past exposure to the risk factor being investigated. The comparison of results between the two groups is expressed as an **odds ratio**. Differential recall of exposure in the two groups, and difficulties in selecting appropriate cases and controls are common sources of **bias** in this type of study (**recall bias, selection bias**). **Berkson's fallacy** is also a known cause of spurious associations found in some studies. Case-control studies are particularly helpful in the study of rare conditions and infectious disease outbreaks. Sometimes called **retrospective study**, since patients who have already been diagnosed are usually used as cases, although some case-control studies are conducted **prospectively**, i.e. using new, rather than existing cases.

Categorical variable

Variable whose values represent different categories or classes of the same feature. Examples are ethnicity, blood group and eye colour, which can also be called **nominal variables**. When the variable has only two categories it is termed **binary** (e.g. sex). If there is an inherent ordering or where a **quantitative variable** has been categorized, it is called an **ordinal variable**.

Cause–effect relationship

Describes the relationship between two factors which are associated, whenever it can be established that one of the factors causes the other. Several criteria must be met (Bradford-Hill criteria, in SACKETT *et al.* 1991; WALD, 1996) before such conclusion can be reached. Essential criteria are: lack of **bias** in the investigation (due to **confounding** or other reasons), small probability of a **type I error** (or small **P-value**) and the demonstration of a temporal relationship (cause precedes effect). Other criteria are the strength of the relationship, the existence of a dose–response relationship, consistency with other studies, and biological plausibility of the hypothesis put forward.

The latter cannot be verified by statistical calculations, but is nonetheless of extreme importance, and should not be ignored if the investigation is to be meaningful.

Censoring

In the context of **follow-up studies**, the **outcome** (e.g. death) of a subject is said to be censored if the same outcome is not observed within the **follow-up period** for that subject. Loss to follow-up frequently leads to censoring since the outcome remains unknown.

Chi-squared (χ^2) test

Significance test for comparing two or more **proportions** from independent groups. It can also be used to test for an association between two **nominal variables** (e.g. ethnicity and blood group) or between a nominal and an **ordinal variable** [e.g. oral cancer (**binary**) and amount of alcohol consumption]. In the latter case the χ-squared test for **trend** should be used. When carrying out the χ-squared test, the observed frequencies (O) are displayed in a **contingency table**, and the **expected frequencies (E)** calculated. This is done for each cell in the table (for Table 1 the cells are a, b, c and d). The test is based on the differences between observed and expected frequencies across the cells: the greater the differences the greater the evidence to reject the **null hypothesis** of no difference (the smaller the **P-value** produced by the test). The test statistic is calculated as follows:

$$\chi^2_{df} = \sum \frac{(O - E)^2}{E}$$

The **statistical significance** of the results also depends on the size of the table, i.e. on the number of categories of the two variables involved, represented by the **degrees of freedom (df)** of the test: the larger the table the greater the differences need to be for statistical significance to be achieved. The **assumptions** for the chi-squared test are **independence** of observations (i.e. each observation coming from a different subject), at least 80% of the cells with expected frequencies greater than five and all cells with expected frequencies greater than one. When these assumptions are not met other tests, such as the **Fisher's exact test**, should be used. The **McNemar's test** is indicated when analysing paired (non-independent) proportions. When the chi-squared test is used with small samples (roughly less than 30) in analysing **two-by-two tables**, a correction (Yates' correction) should be applied to the chi-squared statistic to avoid incorrect results. A worked example is given in Appendix C.

Clinical significance

Magnitude of a treatment effect, expressed in terms such as **relative risk**, **absolute risk difference**, or **number needed to treat**. A decision on clinical significance requires a clinical or public health judgement as to what is a large effect. An effect which is **statistically significant** may nonetheless be too small to warrant any changes in treatment or other policies, in which case the same result is not considered to be clinically significant. The converse can also occur, i.e. clinical significance without statistical significance. This last scenario should be avoided by using study **samples** of appropriate **size**. **Confidence intervals** can help assess the clinical significance of study results (Box 3, p 13).

Clinical trial   Comparative study in which researchers intervene in the natural course of a disease, by administering drugs or other treatments/interventions to at least one of the study groups, and then assessing the effect of the same treatments. The paradigm of clinical trials is the **randomized controlled trial**. POCOCK (1983) gives a full discussion of issues related to clinical trials.

Cluster analysis   **Multivariate method** also referred to as unsupervised pattern recognition (in artificial intelligence language). Profiles for subjects being studied are compared, and subjects who are 'close' together are classified as being in the same cluster or group. The term 'profile' refers to a set of measurements pertaining to a single subject. These may be **repeated measurements** of a single variable (e.g. pain scores over a 5-h period, after 30 min exercise, in patients with arthritis), measurements on a variety of factors (pain, flexibility, depression, haematological parameters), or a combination of both.

Cluster sampling   Method of **sampling** in which groups of subjects are treated as the sampling units, as opposed to simple **random** sampling, where individuals are the sampling units. Typically, entire households, schools or general practices are sampled. If the study in question is a **randomized controlled trial**, all individuals in a particular unit will be given the same treatment or intervention. This is done for practical and ethical reasons. For example, in a study on the relationship between vitamin C supplements and incidence of influenza in school children, parents of children not receiving vitamin C may find it not acceptable that other children in the same school are receiving a potentially beneficial intervention. They may even decide to give vitamin C tablets to their children, which could result in serious contamination of the **control** group. When calculating the **sample size required** in a study where clusters are the sampling units, it is necessary to make adjustments to the formulae commonly used. The *effective sample size* of the study will be less than the total number of individuals in the study.

Coefficient of variation	Measure of the **repeatability** of a measurement method. Calculated by taking repeated measurements with the method in question, and dividing the 'standard deviation of the measurement errors' (see repeatability) by the **mean** of *all* repeated measurements. Sometimes multiplied by 100 and expressed as a percentage. Less ideal if used in situations where the error of the method is not proportional to the magnitude of the measurements. See BLAND (1995).
Cohort	Group of subjects sharing some common characteristic, which is **followed-up** in a research study for a specified period of time. In studies of prognosis, an 'inception cohort' of patients just diagnosed or in the early stages of treatment can give a better **estimate** of the true probability of survival or failure.
Cohort study	Analytical **observational study** which aims to investigate the relationship between an **exposure** or **risk factor** and one or more **outcomes**, by following up two or more **cohorts** over a period of time (**follow-up** or longitudinal study). The level of exposure of each cohort is established at the beginning of the study. Loss to follow-up and surveillance bias (**information bias**) are two common sources of **bias** in this type of study. Sometimes termed **prospective study**.
Collinearity	In the context of **regression**. Collinearity is present when there is perfect association between **predictor variables**, i.e. the predictors in question vary together, and totally 'explain' each other. More frequently, variables explain each other only in part, and are said to be **correlated** or highly correlated (e.g. socioeconomic variables). The presence of highly correlated variables in the same **model** results in unstable regression models. Therefore, the fitting of regression models should be a careful, thorough procedure, especially if carried out in an automated way using a computer package. Exploratory analyses prior to the model fitting can clarify many of the relationships between predictor variables, and between predictor and **outcome variables**.
Conditional logistic regression	**Regression** method for paired **binary** data. A common application of this type of **logistic regression** is the analysis of **case-control studies** where cases and controls have been individually **matched**. An example would be a study where the relationship between use of oral contraceptives and breast cancer is investigated in women aged between 20 and 60 years. Women with breast cancer are individually matched for age with a **control** (since the risk of breast cancer increases with age), which results in paired, non-**independent** data.

Confidence interval (CI)

In the context of **estimation,** a CI is a range of values within which the 'true' **population** parameter is believed to be found, with a given level of confidence. This is a frequently used definition of CIs. In the strict sense, a CI is one of a large number of CIs, all estimating the same population parameter, and all based on study samples of the same size, a given percentage of which *will* contain the true population parameter. The parameters of interest are usually **means, proportions,** differences between means and proportions, **regression coefficients, correlation coefficients, relative risks.** The rationale for calculating CIs is the uncertainty which is always associated with using **samples** to obtain information about the populations from which these samples originate. A single value ('point estimate') is likely to be **inaccurate** so the 95% CI provides additional information about the population value: we can be 95% confident the population value lies within its limits. Different levels of confidence can be placed on a CI, so 90% or 99% CIs can also be calculated. A 99% CI will be wider than the corresponding 95% CI. The width of a CI depends also on the **sample size,** larger samples providing narrower CIs. CIs are extremely useful in assessing the **clinical significance** of a given result. The lower and/ or upper boundaries of a CI may indicate the possibility of important treatment effects in negative trials, or lack of effect in positive trials. Generally, a 95% CI is calculated as follows:

$$95\% \; CI = \text{sample estimate} \pm 1.96 \times SE$$

[In the case of means, this formula applies for large samples. For smaller samples (roughly less than 30) the **standard error (SE)** of the estimate should be multiplied by the critical value of t which can be found in tables of the t-distribution against the appropriate number of **degrees of freedom.**] CIA, by GARDNER *et al.* (1991), is a statistical package for calculating CIs for different estimates. This is the computer version of *Statistics with Confidence,* edited by GARDNER and ALTMAN (1989).

BOX 3

From **Box 1**, p 1.

The 95% CI for the ARD (absolute risk difference) was from 1.5 to 3.4%: for each 1000 AMI patients given aspirin, between 15 and 34 vascular deaths are believed to be prevented (at five weeks), with 95% certainty. Both values are clinically significant and justify a change of treatment policy since the results are not likely to be due to chance ($P < 0.00001$).

Confounding

Error which occurs when groups being compared in a study are different, with regard to important **risk** or **prognostic factors** other than the factor (treatment or **exposure**) under investigation. The results of such a study are likely to be **biased**. For example, if a group of people who exercise regularly and a group of people who do not exercise have an important age difference, then a difference found in **incidence** of heart disease could well be due to one group being older rather than the exercising: age is acting as a confounder, and the effect of exercising on heart disease prevention cannot be properly assessed. **Crude estimates** are not valid under these circumstances and **adjusted estimates** should be obtained instead. Certain **study designs** are more prone to bias via confounding, in particular the **case-control design**, given the difficulty in collecting reliable information on potential confounders. **Randomized trials** take care of this problem (at least in principle) by making groups comparable in relation to known and unknown prognostic factors. The example in Box 4 (ROTHMAN, 1986) illustrates some of the above concepts.

BOX 4

Mann JI et al. (1968). Oral contraceptive use in older women and fatal myocardial infarction. Br Med J **2**: 193–199.

In this study, 153 women with myocardial infarction and 178 controls were investigated for past exposure to oral contraceptives. The crude **odds ratio (OR)** estimate (without taking age into account) was calculated as follows:

	User	Non-user
Cases	39	114
Controls	24	154
OR	2.2	(i.e. 39/24÷114/154 = 39/114÷24/154)

After **stratification** by age group, the results in each age group were:

	Age <40		Age 40–44	
	User	Non-user	User	Non-user
Cases	21	26	18	88
Controls	17	59	7	95
OR	2.8		2.8	

These adjusted OR estimates show that age confounded the assessment of the relationship between oral contraceptives and myocardial infarction in older women. However, the confounding effect of age was not a strong one, given the magnitude of the differences between crude and adjusted ORs. The confounding effect (weakened relationship) occurred because:

1 Age is associated with exposure: 38 out of 123 (31%) of women aged <40 years were 'users', compared to 12% of those aged 40–44 years.

2 There is a greater proportion of women aged <40 years among the controls than among the cases: 43% vs 31%.

Contingency table

Table 1 gives examples of contingency tables. These are used to summarize the association between two **categorical variables**. The rows represent the different levels of one of the variables, and the columns the different levels of the other variable.

Table I Contingency tables

Observational study

		Exposure		
		Yes	No	Total
Outcome	**Yes**	a	b	$a + b$
	No	c	d	$c + d$
	Total	$a + c$	$b + d$	$a + b + c + d$

Clinical trial

		Treatment/intervention		
		Yes	No	Total
Outcome	**Yes**	a	b	$a + b$
	No	c	d	$c + d$
	Total	$a + c$	$b + d$	$a + b + c + d$

The cells contain the observed frequencies resulting from the cross-tabulation of the two variables. These cells are mutually exclusive, where each subject in a study can be in one and only one of the cells. Totals must always be presented. Most commonly, the **chi-squared test** and related methods are appropriate to analyse contingency tables. When carrying out the chi-squared test, **degrees of freedom** are calculated as $(r - 1) \times (c - 1)$, where r is the number of rows and c is the number of columns. When the two variables are **ordinal** (e.g. level of pain and cancer stage), **rank correlation** methods are indicated. When one variable is ordinal and the other is **binary** (e.g. degree of smoking and heart disease), a **trend test** should be used. The **Kruskal–Wallis test** is indicated when one variable is ordinal and the other has three or more categories.

Continuous variable

Quantitative variable which can theoretically take any value within a given range (e.g. height and weight).

Controls

Subjects used in comparative studies to act as the standard against which new treatments or interventions are to be tested (as in **randomized controlled trials**), or against which the risks connected with a particular **exposure** are evaluated (as in **case-control studies**). Controls can be concurrent or historical, depending on whether these subjects are investigated at the same time/place and in the same way as those not acting as controls. **Crossover trials** use just a single group of subjects, where each individual acts as her or his own control.

Correlation	Linear association between two **quantitative** or **ordinal variables**, measured by a **correlation coefficient**. Correlations should only be obtained for **random samples**, and not when the values of one of the variables have been handpicked (e.g. in a laboratory experiment). See ALTMAN (1991) for a discussion of spurious correlations in the literature.
Correlation coefficient	Measure of the linear association between **quantitative** or **ordinal variables**. Can be obtained using **parametric (Pearson's)** or **non-parametric methods (rank correlation)** (Figures 14 and 18, pp 56 and 77). Values taken range from −1 (perfect negative association) to +1 (perfect positive association), with 0 representing lack of linear association. (Note: for rank correlation, it is the linear association between the **ranks** given to the data values of each variable.)
Cost-benefit analysis	Comparison of the costs and **outcomes** of different treatments/interventions when these interventions have different effects, or similar multiple effects of different magnitude. Thus, simple **cost-effectiveness** comparisons are difficult to make, and outcomes and costs are usually translated into their money value. A ratio of money spent (cost value) to money gained (outcome value) can be used to compare different interventions (e.g. a hypertension screening program vs an influenza immunization programme – DRUMMOND 1994, DRUMMOND et al., 1997; the outcomes are prevention of premature death and prevention of days of disability).
Cost-effectiveness analysis	Comparison of the costs and **outcomes** of alternative treatments/ interventions, when these interventions are thought to have the same effect, but not the same magnitude of effect (e.g. kidney transplantation and inpatient dialysis for patients with renal failure – DRUMMOND, 1994; DRUMMOND et al., 1997; the outcome is survival, which can be longer with one treatment than with the other).
Cost-minimization analysis	Comparison of the costs and **outcomes** of alternative treatments/ interventions, when these interventions can be shown to have comparable results or impact (e.g. day-surgery and inpatient surgery for patients with haemorrhoids – DRUMMOND, 1994; DRUMMOND et al., 1997; the outcome is successful correction of the problem).
Cost-utility analysis	Comparison of the costs and **outcomes** of different treatments/ interventions, when these interventions have different effects, or similar

single or multiple effects, of different magnitude. Thus, simple **cost-effectiveness** comparisons are difficult to make, since their impact or importance may not be the same from patient to patient or from situation to situation. This type of analysis allows individual preferences, values and circumstances to be taken into account. Outcomes are translated into their utility value, usually 'quality-adjusted life-years or QALYs'. QALYs are then used to compare the costs of different interventions – DRUMMOND (1994) and DRUMMOND *et al.* (1997).

Cox regression

Regression method for modelling **survival** times. [Also called proportional hazards **model** since it assumes the ratio of the risks (or **hazard ratio, HR**) of the event (e.g. death) at any particular time, between any two groups being compared, to be constant.] The **outcome variable** is whether or not the event of interest has occurred, and if so, after what period of time, if not, the duration of follow-up. The model predicts the hazard or risk of the event in question (commonly death) at any given time. The **predictor variables** are **prognostic factors** as with any other type of regression model. Cox regression can be considered a 'semi-**parametric**' method, since no other **assumptions**, namely about the **distribution** of survival times, are made. See ALTMAN (1991) for further discussion. Box 5 gives an example of Cox regression, using a ficticious cancer drug trial.

BOX 5

STATA Corporation (1997). Cancer drug trial data, in *STATA Statistical Software release 5*. College Station, TX: STATA Corporation (used with permission).

The results presented are for a cancer drug trial where 48 patients were randomized either to the treatment group (28 patients) or to the control group (20 patients). Age of the participants ranged from 47 to 67 years, and was categorized into five-year intervals. Time to death is measured in months. Some observations are **censored** (patient alive at the end of study period or lost to follow-up). Thirty-one deaths were observed over 744 person-months at risk (see **person-time at risk**).

The Cox regression analysis yielded the following results:

	HR	95% CI	P-value
1 For the effect of the drug	0.105	0.043 to 0.256	<0.0005
2 For the effect of age	1.76	1.225 to 2.543	0.002

Interpretation:

1 The death hazard in the drug group is 0.105 that in the control group.

2 For each five-year increase in age, the death hazard is expected to increase by a factor of 1.76.

See also **Kaplan–Meier method** and **log rank test**.

Cronbach's alpha	Measure of the **reliability** of a composite rating scale, made up of several items or variables. Psychological and mental health tests are common examples of this type of scale.

Crossover design	Study design for a **clinical trial** in which all patients are given the two or more treatments under investigation, such that each patient acts as her or his own **control**. As a result, the **sample size required** is smaller than with a **parallel design** (where different groups are given different treatments), given the lesser degree of **variability** within the same subjects. **Randomization** is used to assign the *order* in which the treatments are to be administered (Box 6), mainly to avoid **period effects**. Main limitations of this type of design are the fact that it cannot be used with diseases which can be cured, with acute conditions, or when treatment periods are too long, as patients may be prone to **drop-out**. There is also a potential for **carry-over** of treatment effects from one period into the next, resulting in **treatment-period interaction**. The latter should be given careful consideration in the planning stages of a trial so that it can be avoided by introducing appropriate **wash-out periods**. In the presence of a treatment-period interaction, data for the second period are usually discarded. The result is a parallel design trial which is likely not to be sufficiently large to ensure adequate **power**. See POCOCK (1983) for further discussion.

BOX 6
Weinshenker B *et al.* (1992). A double-blind, randomized crossover trial of pemoline in fatigue associated with multiple sclerosis. *Neurology* **42**: 1468–1471.
Total number of patients = 46
Five patients dropped out due to exacerbation of their condition
23 randomized to receive pemoline first
18 randomized to receive placebo first
Wash-out period: two weeks

	First period (four weeks)		Second period (four weeks)
N = 23	A	→	B
N = 18	B	→	A

Cross-overs	Subjects participating in a **clinical trial**, who, for some reason, do not take or receive the treatment to which they were allocated, but instead, take or receive the alternative treatment in the trial. **Intention-to-treat analysis** is recommended to minimize the **biases** which result from these protocol breaches.

Cross-sectional study

Type of **observational study**. As opposed to a **follow-up study**, subjects are observed on just one occasion. It is thus very difficult to infer a **cause–effect relationship** from such a **study design**. Descriptive cross-sectional studies are usually referred to as **surveys**. Common problems with this type of study are the selection of the study **sample**, **random sampling** being the only way of ensuring a representative sample, non-response and **volunteer bias**, all leading to **selection bias**. A cross-sectional design gives **estimates** of **prevalence** (how much disease exists) rather than **incidence** (how many new cases develop in a certain period of time).

Crude estimates

Estimates which are obtained without controlling for **confounding** factors, as opposed to **adjusted estimates**. If confounding is suspected in a study, crude estimates may be misleading when making comparisons. For example, different **populations** often have different age structures. Thus, direct comparisons made between these populations (e.g. mortality from heart disease) will be **biased** if age is not taken into account. See Box 4 (p 14) for an example of crude estimates.

Cumulative hazard

In the context of **survival analysis**, it summarizes the risk of an event over a specified period of time or **follow-up period**. The cumulative hazard or failure rate is calculated from the **Kaplan–Meier estimate** of cumulative survival $[S(t)]$ using the following formula:

$$H(t) = -\log S(t)$$

Cumulative meta-analysis

Special **meta-analysis** technique which integrates the results from individual studies, as these studies are carried out and results become available. The graphical display of a cumulative meta-analysis shows the pooled **effect sizes** of all studies carried out up to a particular point in time, going from the first study (at the top) to the last (at the bottom), which includes all other studies. Since with each additional step data from a new study are included, the 'sample size' increases and the **confidence interval** for the pooled **estimate** becomes narrower, reflecting increasing certainty. Figure 5 shows a cumulative meta-analysis, corresponding to the graph presented in Figure 9, p 42 (SMITH et al., 1993, Figure 5).

Decision analysis

Systematic way of reaching a medical decision, based on evidence from research. This information is translated into probabilities, and incorporated in diagrams or decision trees which direct the clinician through a succession of possible scenarios, actions and **outcomes**. An important concept in decision analysis is that of patient's utilities, i.e. of the relative value of each

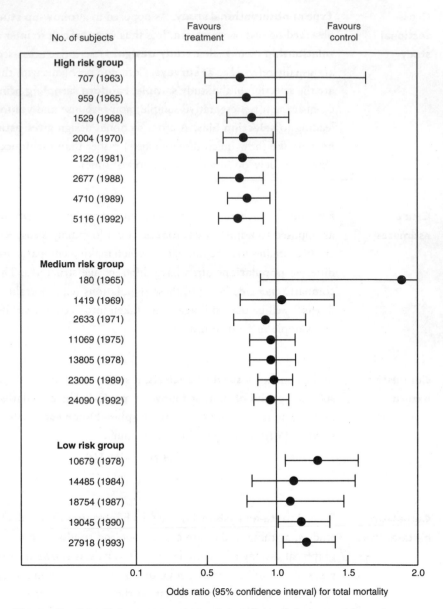

Figure 5 Cumulative meta-analysis of the effect of cholesterol lowering on total mortality, in relation to risk of death from coronary heart disease per 1000 PYAR [reproduced with permission from Smith, Song and Sheldon (1993). Cholestrol lowering and mortality: the importance of considering initial level of risk. *Br Med J* **306**: 1367–1373].

outcome for an individual patient. Decision trees are also used in **diagnostic testing**. Figure 6 shows an example of a decision tree (DAWSON-SAUNDERS and TRAPP, 1994, Figure 14-3, p 253, reproduced with permission). The starting point of the decision tree is a specific medical problem, and the outcomes of the different possible courses of action (squares) are given by the circles. An expected utility (EU, ranging from 0 – no value to 100 – ideal outcome) is attached to each of these outcomes. The probabilities for the different outcomes, shown on the branches of the tree, are extracted from the results of previous research. The tree is analysed starting from the outcomes, and working 'back' the expected utilities of the different courses of action. In this example, and given the value or utility attached to each outcome, surgery is the preferred course of action.

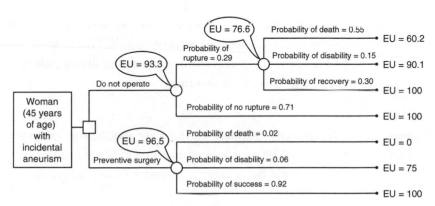

Figure 6 Decision tree for aneurysms with probabilities and utilities included [with permission from van Crevel H, Habbema J, Braakman R (1986). Decision analysis of the management of incidental intracranial saccular aneurysms. *Neurology* **36**: 1335–1339].

Degrees of freedom (df)

Measure used in many **significance tests** and other statistical procedures, which reflects the **sample size(s)** of the study group(s) used in an investigation. The larger the sample size(s), the greater the **power** to prove a given result as **statistically significant**, i.e. not likely to be due to chance. For **categorical** data, test results depend also on the size of **contingency tables** used to summarize the association between two variables. Tables with excessive numbers of categories may have reduced power, compared to smaller tables (fewer observations in each cell). Sample and table sizes are expressed in terms of degrees of freedom. The way these are calculated depends on the statistical test in question.

Detection bias

See **selection bias**.

Detection rate

See **sensitivity**.

Deviance

Statistic used to assess the goodness of **fit** or appropriateness of **regression models** fitted by the method of **maximum likelihood** (in fact, the badness of fit, since the greater the deviance the worse the fit of a model). Models which have many **predictor variables** may be simplified, provided important information is not lost in the process. This is tested by the difference in deviance between any two nested models being compared (**likelihood ratio test**): the smaller the difference in deviance the smaller the impact of the variables removed.

Diagnostic tests

Clinical, laboratory, radiological or other tests, which are carried out for the purpose of establishing an actual diagnosis. These tests are usually motivated by the presence of signs and/or symptoms of disease, which makes diagnostic testing different from **screening**.

Discrete variable

Quantitative variable which, unlike **continuous variables**, can only take certain values, usually integers (e.g. number of children, number of patients in a practice list, number of asthma episodes in a year).

Discriminant analysis

Multivariate method of classifying subjects into known groups, on the basis of their profile of measurements (e.g. symptoms). It is a form of computerized diagnosis, also known as supervised pattern recognition (in artificial intelligence language). Linear discriminant analysis and **logistic regression** are the methods commonly used for this purpose. In addition to finding a discriminant rule or **model**, it is important to assess its performance, i.e. the misclassification rate or proportion of subjects incorrectly classified. Ideally, an **independent** sample of subjects should be used to estimate this error rate. The search for the best sub-set of **predictor** or explanatory variables can be done by a **stepwise** procedure.

Distributions

Probability distributions are used to calculate the probability of different values occurring, under various assumed distributions of known theoretical form: **normal** (Figure 10, p 46), binomial, Poisson. These distributions are defined mathematically by one or more parameters. **Parametric** statistical methods rely quite strongly on the **assumption** that the data have an empirical distribution which approximates the theoretical ones. For **quantitative variables**, which are frequently required to have a normal distribution, this can be checked by looking at a **histogram** depicting the shape of its relative frequency distribution (Figure 10), or at a **normal plot**

(Figures 11 and 12, p 47). When the required assumptions cannot be met, it is possible to resort to data **transformations** or to **non-parametric methods**.

Double blind   See **blinding**.

Drop-outs   See **withdrawals**.

Dummy variable

In the context of **regression**, dummy or indicator variables are created whenever it is necessary to incorporate a **categorical variable** into a **model**. If this step is not taken, a categorical variable such as blood group, whose levels are coded with labels say, from 1 to 4 (O, A, B, AB), will be interpreted as a **quantitative variable**, and a numerical meaning will be given to the labels. In the above example, four new dummy variables are created:

Patient	Blood group	Dummy variables			
		BG1	BG2	BG3	BG4
1	1 (O)	1	0	0	0
2	3 (B)	0	0	1	0
3	4 (AB)	0	0	0	1
4	1 (O)	1	0	0	0
5	2 (A)	0	1	0	0
...					

See **analysis of covariance** (Box 2, p 3) for an example of the use and interpretation of dummy variables in regression models.

Dunnett's correction

Procedure which gives corrected **P-values** when performing **multiple significance tests**. Used when the comparisons are made between the different levels of a **categorical variable** and the baseline level for the same variable. *P*-values are multiplied by the number of comparisons made, but **sample sizes** are also taken into account.

Effect size

Standardized **estimate** of a treatment effect (e.g. difference between two **means** or **proportions**), used in the context of **meta-analyses** when the outcomes analysed in the different studies are related but not the same (e.g. flexibility and pain in patients with arthritis). To obtain the effect size, the estimate is divided by the **standard deviation** of the measurements (means), or proportions ($\sqrt{[p(1-p)]}$), where p is the average of the two proportions. Effect sizes are also calculated when using nomograms for **power** calculations (see Box 21, p 61).

Estimates **Summary measures** calculated from **samples**. Estimates can be **means, proportions, regression coefficients, relative risks**, etc. These can be more precisely termed 'point estimates'. Estimates are used to make inferences about **target populations**, whose 'true' values or parameters are not known. Estimates should be quoted with the corresponding **standard errors (SE)**, usually translated into **confidence intervals** ('interval estimates') for ease of interpretation.

Excess See **relative risk reduction**.
relative risk

Expected as opposed to observed frequencies (O). In a **contingency table** they are the
frequencies numbers or frequencies expected in each cell, under the **assumption** that the
(E) **null hypothesis** is true, i.e. of no relationship between **exposure** (or treatment) and **outcome**. For each cell, they are calculated as follows:

$$E = \frac{\text{row total} \times \text{column total}}{\text{grand total}}$$

In Table 1, for example, the expected frequency in the first cell (a) is: $\{(a + c) \times (a + b)\} \div (a + b + c + d)$.

Experimental See **clinical trial**.
study

Explanatory See **predictor variable**.
variable

Exposure Factor (including treatments and interventions) which is thought to be associated with the development (**risk factor**) or prevention (protective factor) of a given condition or **outcome**.

F-test or **variance**-ratio test. **Significance test** used in **analysis of variance** as a method of assessing whether the **population means** of several groups are similar, by comparing the between-groups and within-groups **variability**.

Under the **null hypothesis** of no difference among the populations being compared, these two quantities are the same and their ratio (*F*-statistic) is equal to one. The *F*-**distribution** (which is followed by the *F*-statistic when the null hypothesis is true) has two sets of **degrees of freedom**: the number of groups -1 (between-groups), and the total number of observations minus the number of groups (within-groups). When comparing two **independent** groups, the *F*-test yields the same result as the unpaired **t-test**. In **regression** analysis, the *F*-test can be used to test the joint significance of all variables in a **model**. Models which are related, where one model is an extension of the other (nested), can be compared using the *F*-test.

Factor analysis

Multivariate method that analyses **correlations** between sets of observed measurements, with the view to estimate the number of different factors which explain these correlations. For example, correlations between components of a composite intelligence rating scale are inferred to arise from the fact that they (the sub-scales or sets of measurements) are all measures of intelligence (the factor). An exploratory factor analysis looks at these correlations, assesses the number of factors which might need to be postulated to provide an explanation for the correlations, and decides what variables might be indicators of what factors. A confirmatory factor analysis assesses whether a set of correlations can be adequately explained by a factor **model** specified *a priori*.

Factorial design

Study design for a **clinical trial**, which allows two or more different treatments to be compared with each other and with a **control**. In a 2×2 factorial design patients are divided into four groups, each receiving either the control treatment, treatment A, treatment B or both treatments A and B. This design allows the investigation of several hypotheses simultaneously, including that of synergism or **interaction** between the two treatments (Box 7). See POCOCK (1983) for examples and discussion.

BOX 7

From **Box 1**, p 1.

In the ISIS-2 trial, patient randomization was first to streptokinase vs placebo, and then to aspirin vs placebo, resulting in four treatment groups. The arrows represent the different comparisons made possible by the study design:

		Streptokinase Yes	No	Total
Aspirin	Yes	4292	4295	8587
	No	4300	4300	8600
	Total	8592	8595	17,187

False negative rate	See **sensitivity**.

False positive rate	See **specificity**.

Fisher's exact test **Significance test** for comparing **proportions**. Used as an alternative to the **chi-squared test**, whenever the **assumption** regarding **expected frequencies** is not met or the total sample size is too small (<30). The test gives exact probabilities (**P-values**) under a special **distribution** (the hypergeometric distribution).

Fit (goodness of) Measure of how well a theoretical **distribution** or a specified **model** fit a set of data. It is based on the comparison of observed and **expected frequencies**. Many **significance tests** such as the **chi-squared test** are in fact goodness-of-fit tests. Common applications of goodness-of-fit tests are the assessment of **normality** and the **Hosmer and Lemeshow chi-squared test**, used in the context of **logistic regression**, to assess the predictive ability of a given model.

Fixed effects As opposed to **random effects**. Term used in the context of **meta-analysis**, when results from several studies are combined (producing a single **estimate**) by taking a weighted average of the individual results, usually according to study size. It is accepted that this combined estimate can be applied to any subjects from any of the **target populations** represented by the individual studies. The assumption is that the underlying 'true' population parameters are the same in each of these studies. Tests of **heterogeneity** are used to decide on the choice of a random or a fixed effects model. In the context of **analysis of variance (ANOVA)**, the term is used to describe factors all of whose categories may be identified (e.g. gender, ethnicity, blood group), in contrast to random effects factors (e.g. patients A, D and E, as opposed to patients B, C and F).

Follow-up period Length of time subjects are kept under observation in a particular study. A distinction is sometimes made between the actual follow-up period and the accrual period in which patients are recruited to the study. In a trial where the aim is to compare **survival** times, it is particularly important to count follow-up from **randomization**, and not from the actual time treatments are given. For example, if patients are randomized to receive either medical (drugs) or surgical treatment for the management of unstable angina, patients having surgery may have to wait longer for their treatment. Thus, if follow-up time is counted from beginning of treatment, patients receiving the medical treatment are given a clear advantage.

Follow-up study

Longitudinal or **prospective study**. Study in which information is collected by following subjects over a period of time, thus allowing temporal relationships to be investigated.

Gaussian distribution

See **normal distribution**.

Geometric mean

Anti-log of a **mean** calculated from observations which have been **transformed** to a log scale. **Quantitative variables** which display a positive **skew** (i.e. with more observations with lower values than with higher values) may sometimes have a **lognormal distribution**, i.e. their logarithmic transform has a **normal distribution** (e.g. serum triglycerides). **Parametric methods** of **estimation** (e.g. calculation of a simple arithmetic mean) and/ or **significance testing** can be applied to the log values, and the results backtransformed to their original scale. Figure 7 shows the distribution of length of hospital stay, for a particular type of surgery, as being positively skewed. The mean and **median** for the original values are marked on the graph (A and B), as well as the geometric mean (C). The geometric mean is closer to the median, both being approximately two days shorter than the arithmetic mean and more representative of the majority of observations.

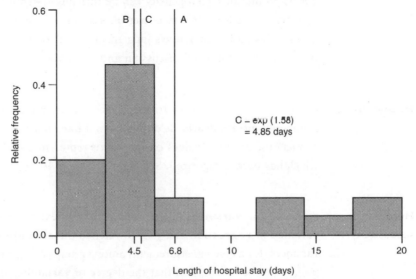

Figure 7 Arithmetic and geometric means for a positively skewed distribution.

Gold standard — In the context of **diagnostic testing**, it refers to a **valid (1)** diagnostic tool which consistently gives the correct diagnosis (i.e. **reliable** and **accurate**). In practice, gold standards are rarely 100% accurate. They are simply the best method of diagnosis according to current dogma. Gold standard tests are often invasive or expensive diagnostic methods, but can be used in studies to assess the performance (**sensitivity, specificity**) of simpler and/or cheaper methods.

Hazard ratio (HR) — Measure of **relative risk** used in **survival** studies. It is calculated as follows:

$$HR = \frac{O_1/E_1}{O_2/E_2}$$

where O_1 is the observed number of subjects with the event in group 1; E_1 is the **expected** number of subjects with the event in group 1, under the hypothesis (**null hypothesis**) that the two groups being compared experience the same event hazard (i.e. the overall hazard applied to the total number of subjects in this subgroup); O_2 and E_2 as above, for group 2. An HR of 1 suggests the hazard or risk of the event is the same in the two groups being compared. An HR greater than 1 suggests group 1 is more likely to experience the event. The opposite is true for an HR less than 1. See Box 5 (p 17) for an example and interpretation.

Hetero-geneity — or lack of homogeneity. Term usually employed in the context of **meta-analyses**, when the results or **estimates** from individual studies appear to have different magnitude, or even different sign or direction. In the presence of marked heterogeneity a single summary of these individual results should not be produced. Heterogeneity can be formally tested using special tests. However, these are not very powerful and can be misleading. Heterogeneity is best assessed by using one's judgement. See Thompson (in CHALMERS and ALTMAN, 1995) for a full discussion and references.

Histogram — Graphical display of the distribution of a **quantitative variable**, most commonly **interval/ratio**. It differs from a **bar chart** in that the bars are contiguous, since the values on the x-axis represent a numerical variable which has been categorized. See Figure 10 on p 46.

Homo-scedasticity — or equality of **variances**. Term used in the context of **t-tests, analysis of variance** or **regression** analysis, to refer to the **assumption** of equal variances (for a given measurement) among groups being compared (Figure 4, p 8), or to the assumption that the degree of **variability** in the **outcome variable** is about the same for all values of a **predictor variable**.

Hosmer and Lemeshow χ^2 statistic	Statistic which assesses the **predictive** ability of a **logistic regression model**. To perform the test, the probability of a particular event is computed for each observation, using the model obtained. Observations are then grouped into 'probability or risk of event categories' (e.g. 0–10%, 10%+, 20%+, ..., 90%+) and a $r \times 2$ **contingency table** is produced with the columns representing the outcome (yes/no type) and the rows representing 'risk of event categories' as indicated above. The cells of this table contain the observed frequencies for each cross-tabulation. The test statistic is computed from the differences between observed and **expected frequencies** in each cell. A **chi-squared test** on $r - 2$ **degrees of freedom** tests whether or not predicted values are close to observed values (r is the number of risk of event categories). Small **P-values** indicate poor predictive models.
Incidence	as opposed to **prevalence**. Measure of the number of *new* cases of a disease, occurring during a specified period of time. It can be expressed as **incidence rate** or **incidence risk**.
Incidence rate	Measure of morbidity or disease occurrence. Number of new cases of a disease during a specified period of time, with reference to the **person-time at risk** during the same period (note: the denominator is 'time', not 'people'). Usually multiplied by 1000 and expressed per 1000 person-time at risk (or, if the event is rare, per 10 000 or 100 000).
Incidence risk	Measure of morbidity or disease occurrence. Number of new cases of a disease during a specified period of time, with reference to the number of persons at risk of contracting the disease at the beginning of the same period. Usually expressed as a percentage. For rare diseases, the **incidence rate** and the incidence risk will be approximately the same (provided average length of **follow-up** is similar).
Independence	of observations. Two observations or measurements made on the same subject or unit (or on individually **matched** subjects) are said to be paired (not independent from each other). This should be taken into account when carrying out data analyses, since independence is an **assumption** required by many **statistical tests**. In simple cases, non-independence is dealt with by using tests such as the **paired t-test** or the **McNemar's test**, but in more complex cases, when there are several dimensions to the pairing, **summary statistics** or formal methods for **repeated measurements** should be employed.

Information bias	General type of bias which can occur in all types of **study design**, due to systematic errors in measuring **exposures** or responses (**outcomes**), which result in misclassification. Information bias can be caused by inadequate questionnaires (tiresome, difficult or biased questions), observer or interviewer errors (lack of **blinding**; surveillance bias due to differential follow-up of exposed and non-exposed in a **follow-up study**), respondent errors (recall bias due to different memory of past exposures between cases and controls in a **case-control study**; lack of blinding; fear or embarrassment), and instrument errors (e.g. a **diagnostic test** with poor performance).
Intention-to-treat analysis (ITT)	In the context of **randomized controlled trials**. In this type of study, patients are expected to receive the treatments to which they were allocated, but may sometimes **drop-out** or be **withdrawn** from a trial. Some patients ('**cross-overs**') receive treatments other than the ones to which they were **randomized**. To minimize the **bias** arising from these situations, patients should be analysed in the groups to which they were randomized. Including these patients in the treatment group they actually received, or ignoring them altogether, may result in severe bias, and may even lead to spurious reversal of treatment effects.
Interaction	An interaction between two or more factors or variables is said to exist if the effect of one variable is not constant across levels of the other. For example, smoking and obesity are risk factors for several diseases. A possible scenario is for the effect of one of them, say smoking, to be greater among obese than non-obese people. Thus, adding to the independent effects of each of these two risk factors, there is a 'penalty' for being both a smoker and overweight, the end effect being greater than the sum of the two effects. In this situation the two **risk factors** have a synergistic effect. In other situations risk factors can be antagonistic, their simultaneous presence resulting in an end effect which is smaller than the sum of the independent effects. [In **regression** analysis, a **model** with two main effects which interact with each other can be written as: $$\hat{y} = \alpha + \beta_1 x_1 + \beta_2 x_2 + \beta_3 x_1 x_2$$ where β_3 represents the **regression coefficient** for the interaction term. This will normally be positive if the interaction is synergistic or negative if it is antagonistic. See **multiple regression** for an explanation of the model. See also Box 8 (and Box 2, Figure 1, pp 3 and 4), for an example.]
Intercept	In the context of **regression models**, the intercept is a constant value, specific to any given model, which represents the estimated value of the **outcome variable** when the **predictor(s)** is (are) equal to zero.

BOX 8
From **Box 2**, p 3.
Another hypothesis in the risk factors for osteoporosis study is that the effect of smoking on bone density (study units) is different for postmenopausal and premenopausal women. The assessment of this interaction between menopausal status and smoking gives the following results:
1 Effect of menopausal status among non-smokers: On average, 4.68 lower for postmenopausal women. **2** Effect of smoking among premenopausal women: On average, 0.36 higher for smokers. **3** Effect of menopausal status and smoking: On average, 6.39 lower in postmenopausal and smoking women, compared to premenopausal and non-smoking women (the simple sum of the main effects is $-4.32 = -4.68 + 0.36$).
The regression equation can be written in this way: Bone density $= (42.7) - 4.68 * MENO + 0.36 * SMOKE - 2.07 * MENO * SMOKE$ (the intercept is in parentheses). Note: MENO and SMOKE are **dummy variables**, taking the value of 1 for postmenopausal women and smokers, and 0 for premenopausal women and non-smokers. See LAW *et al.* (1997) for full results.

Interim analyses

In the context of **clinical trials,** interim analyses are carried out before the end of the study period, in order to assess whether the accumulating data are beginning to demonstrate a beneficial effect of one treatment over the other, with sufficient certainty. This can avoid having extra patients randomized to an inferior treatment. One problem with interim analyses is the increased risk of false positive findings (due to **multiple significance testing**). Sequential designs – group or continuous – are used to deal with this problem. In the case of group sequential designs, and depending on the number of interim analyses planned, nominal significance levels (constant or varying) are specified so that the overall chance of a **type I error** is kept at an acceptable level. Interim analyses raise many problems, and should always be carefully planned before commencement of a study. See POCOCK (1983) for examples and discussion.

Interquartile range (IQR)

Measure of the **variability** of a set of measurements. It is the interval delimited by the 25th and the 75th **percentiles** (also called lower and upper **quartiles**), and comprises 50% of the observations in a variable (Figure 4, p 8). Used to describe data when the **standard deviation** is not an appropriate measure of variability. The IQR is a **robust** measure in that it is not influenced by extreme observations.

Interval variable	**Quantitative variable** which does not possess a true zero, and which allows negative values. For these variables, unlike for **ratio variables**, the ratio between two values has a different value depending on which scale measurements are made. A well-known example of an interval variable is temperature, measured in degrees Fahrenheit or centigrade. A 10% increase in temperature from, say, 50°F to 55°F does not represent a 10% increase on the centigrade scale: it represents a 28% increase from 10°C to 12.8°C.
Intraclass correlation coefficient (ICC)	Measure of **reliability** or agreement for **quantitative** measurements. Used when replicate measurements have no time sequence (e.g. two white blood cell counts made on the same blood sample). The ICC is calculated using a similar but modified procedure to that used to calculate the **Pearson's correlation coefficient** (DUNN and EVERITT, 1995). Like the latter, the ICC has an ideal value of 1, but the ICC is more appropriate than the Pearson's correlation coefficient for assessing agreement. When the measurement in question can take only two values or categories, the ICC is equivalent to the *kappa* **statistic**.
Jackknifing	Method of validating or assessing the **fit** or appropriateness of a **model**, using the same **sample** which was used to derive the model, as opposed to using an **independent** sample. When assessing the fit of a model, the **residuals** are analysed in a number of ways. To use the residuals from a given model to assess the goodness-of-fit of the same model leads to over-optimistic results. Thus, each residual is calculated from a model which includes all but its corresponding observation. Jackknifed residuals are sometimes called studentized residuals.
Kaplan–Meier method	Method of determining **survival** probability over a period of time, in which probabilities are calculated at the exact points in time where an event of interest has occurred in the study group(s). This information can be used to construct a survival curve, in which the probability of survival remains the same between events, only dropping to coincide with the occurrence of a new event, thus giving the appearance of 'steps' (Figure 8). This is the graphical display of the data analysed in **Cox regression** (Box 5, p 17) – cancer drug trial; here, age is not taken into account. **Censored** observations should ideally be marked on the curve at the times at which they occur. The number of subjects still at risk can be shown at regular time intervals (usually along the x-axis). The method can be used to calculate an **estimate** of cumulative survival, which is used to compute the **cumulative hazard rate**. The survival curves of two or more separate groups can be formally compared

using the **log rank test**. The Kaplan–Meier method differs from the **life table** method in which the 'time' variable is grouped. See ALTMAN (1991) for further discussion.

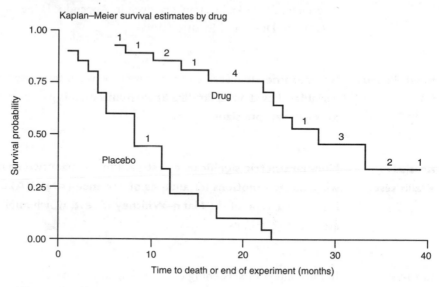

Figure 8   Kaplan–Meier survival curve: cancer drug trial.

kappa statistic (κ)   Measure of agreement for **categorical variables**. It can be used to assess the extent of agreement between two (or more) raters, or between two alternative classification or diagnostic methods. As with the coefficient of **reliability (R)**, κ measures chance-corrected proportional agreement, i.e. the **proportion** of agreement over and above that which might be expected by chance alone:

$$\kappa = \frac{\text{observed agreement} - \text{chance agreement}}{1 - \text{chance agreement}}$$

$$= 1 - \frac{\text{observed disagreement}}{\text{chance-expected disagreement}}$$

Chance agreement is calculated using the method to calculate **expected frequencies** for **contingency tables**. The expected frequencies for cells denoting agreement can then be added up and divided by the total number of observations to give the proportion of agreement which is attributed to chance. κ takes the value of one when there is perfect agreement; zero represents agreement no better than by chance alone, and negative values, agreement worse than expected by chance. With **ordinal variables** the weighted *kappa* statistic can be calculated (ALTMAN, 1991). A common and wrong practice is to test for an association when measuring agreement. This two concepts are not the same, so methods such as the **chi-squared test** or **rank correlation** are not appropriate. *kappa* is dependent on the proportion of subjects in each category and also the **bias** between raters (or methods), i.e. the degree of disagreement between the raters in a study. Thus, it is difficult to give precise values of κ which reflect poor, moderate or good agreement. A worked example is given in Appendix D. See also ALTMAN (1991) and DUNN and EVERITT (1995).

Kendall's tau (τ)	**Non-parametric** measure of association between **quantitative** or **ordinal variables**. Based on **ranks** (like **Spearman's ρ**), it is particularly appropriate for small **sample sizes**.
Kruskal–Wallis test	**Non-parametric significance test** used to compare two or more groups when the **assumptions** for **analysis of variance (ANOVA)** cannot be met. It is an extension of the **Mann–Whitney U-test**, which applies when there are only two groups.
Lead-time bias	In the context of **screening** or early diagnosis, type of **bias** which is caused by detection of disease at a presymptomatic stage, without, however, the possibility of offering a better treatment than that which can be offered to symptomatic patients. When length of survival is **estimated**, patients diagnosed at an earlier stage appear to have longer survival compared to patients diagnosed after developing symptoms. However, this can be a spurious finding, indicative only of the 'zero-time shift' in the time of diagnosis. This is one of the reasons why evidence of the effectiveness of screening programmes must come from **randomized controlled trials** (SACKETT *et al.*, 1991).
Least squares	Method frequently used in **regression** analysis, to find the line of best fit, i.e. the line (or **model**) which best describes the relationship between a **quantitative outcome** and one or more **predictor variables**. The method seeks to minimize the sum of squared **residuals** (i.e. vertical distances from each observation to the regression line). These are used to assess the goodness-of-**fit** of regression models.
Length-time bias	In the context of **screening** or early diagnosis, type of **bias** which results from the preferential diagnosis of disease in patients with long preclinical stages of disease (e.g. slow growing tumours). Because of the positive association between duration of preclinical and clinical stages of disease, early diagnosis may sometimes appear to lead to longer survival. This is one of the reasons why evidence of the effectiveness of screening programmes must come from **randomized controlled trials** (SACKETT *et al.*, 1991).

Life expectancy

Average length of **survival** from beginning of **follow-up**. Calculated using a **life table** as:

$$\text{Life expectancy} = \frac{1}{2} + \sum(\text{number of time units in interval}$$
$$\times \text{cumulative chance of survival})$$

where $\sum$ represents summation.

Life table

Table where the **survival** (or failure) experience of a group of people or **cohort**, over a **follow-up period**, is recorded. The following information is presented (KIRKWOOD, 1988): (1) time, which is commonly expressed as time from beginning of follow-up, or as age. Time is divided into intervals, and for each time interval (or age group) a number of summaries can be obtained: (2) number alive at the beginning of interval (or number in each age group). The number alive is the number at risk before correcting for losses to follow-up; (3) number of events (e.g. death) during the interval; (4) number lost to follow-up during each time interval; (5) number at risk is then calculated as:

number at the beginning $-$ (number lost/2)

(6) risk of dying (or of any other event) during each time interval, calculated as:

number of deaths/number at risk

(7) chance of surviving a given time interval calculated as:

1 $-$ risk of dying during the interval

(8) cumulative chance of surviving from beginning of follow-up, which is:

cumulative chance of survival in previous intervals
$\times$ chance of surviving present interval.

The cumulative chance of surviving the various time intervals can then be used to construct a survival curve. It can also be used to calculate **life expectancy**.

Likelihood ratio test

Significance test used in the context of **Cox** (regression for survival data), **logistic** (regression for proportions) and **Poisson regression** (regression for counts and rates). Often used to assess the **statistical significance** of one or more **predictor variables** in a **model** or equation. The test statistic used here is the **deviance**.

Likelihood ratios (LR)

In the context of **diagnostic testing**. Table 2 shows the layout of the results of a hypothetical diagnostic test. Several quantities can be estimated from such a table: **sensitivity**, **specificity** and the test **predictive values**. The

Table 2 Layout of results from a dichotomous diagnostic test

		Disease		
		Present	**Absent**	**Total**
Test result	**Positive**	a	b	$a + b$
	Negative	c	d	$c + d$
	Total	$a + c$	$b + d$	$a + b + c + d$

likelihood ratio expresses how likely it is to find a positive test result in a patient with the disease in question, in comparison with the likelihood of finding the positive result in a patient without the condition:

$$\text{LR} = \frac{\text{likelihood of } + \text{ve test result among diseased}}{\text{likelihood of } + \text{ve test result among non-diseased}} = \frac{a/(a+c)}{b/(b+d)}$$

For a negative test result, the LR expresses the likelihood of finding this test result in patients with the condition relative to the likelihood of the same test result in patients without the condition:

$$\text{LR} = \frac{\text{likelihood of } - \text{ve test result among diseased}}{\text{likelihood of } - \text{ve test result among non-diseased}} = \frac{c/(a+c)}{d/(b+d)}$$

Likelihood ratios do not have the drawbacks of the other quantities mentioned above: they are not affected by changes in the **prevalence** of disease and they can be used when the test results are grouped into more than two categories. Another desirable property is the fact that they can be converted into the **posttest probability** of disease by knowledge of the **pretest probability** of disease (see also Box 20, p 60). Box 9 presents a nomogram for obtaining posttest probabilities directly from pretest probabilities and LRs.

Log rank test   **Significance test** for comparing the **survival** experience of two or more distinct groups, as expressed by their survival curves. It is a special application of the **Mantel–Haenszel chi-squared test**, where an overall comparison of the groups is performed by summarizing the significance of the differences in survival in each of the time intervals which form the **follow-up period**, thus producing a single test statistic. The number of **degrees of freedom** for the test is the number of groups minus 1. The test can be adjusted for **confounders**, but, in this situation, regression methods for survival data (**Cox regression**) may be preferable. A log rank test for **trend** can also be performed. See Box 10 for an example.

BOX 9

Sackett D, Richardson W, Rosenberg W, Haynes R (1997). *Evidence-based medicine; how to practice and teach EBM.* Churchill Livingstone (reproduced with permission).

The Fagan Likelihood Ratio nomogram:

A straight line is drawn through the values for pre-test probability and LR, and the post-test probability can be read off. For example, if PRE is 30% and LR is 10, POST is just above 80%.

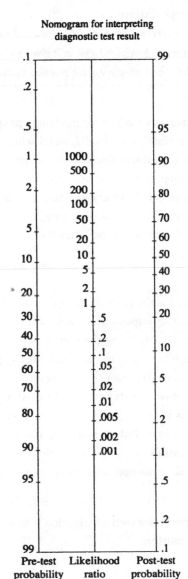

Nomogram for interpreting diagnostic test result

Pre-test probability — Likelihood ratio — Post-test probability

Adapted with permission from Fagan TJ (1975). Nomogram from Bayes' theorem (c). *N Engl J Med* **293**: 257.

BOX 10		
Log-rank test for equality of survivor functions (**Figure 8**, Kaplan–Meier survival curves):		
	Events (death)	
Treatment	Observed (O)	Expected (E)
Drug	12	23.75
Placebo	19	7.25
Total	31	31.00

χ^2 statistic$_{(df=1)}$ = 28.27; $P < 0.00005$.

Interpretation:

The difference between observed and expected number of deaths in each of the treatment groups is large, and gives a highly significant P-value: the drug appears to be more effective than placebo in improving survival.

Logistic regression

Regression method for modelling **proportions**, i.e. **categorical outcomes**. The method is especially useful when dealing with **confounding**, or when assessing **interactions**, with the advantage that **quantitative predictor variables** can also be included in **models**. The **outcome variable** in logistic regression is a **binary variable** (yes/no; alive/dead). The predicted outcome however, is not a binary variable or a proportion, but the logit transformation of the latter (i.e. the natural logarithm of the **odds**):

$$\text{Logit} = \log_e[\text{odds}] = \log_e\left[\frac{p}{1-p}\right]$$

where p is the probability of the event in question. This prevents models from predicting impossible values for a proportion or probability, i.e. outside the range 0 to 1. Using the logit it is possible to work out the predicted probability (p) of the outcome for any given individual. Results from logistic regression are frequently presented as **odds ratios (OR)**. If data are individually **matched, conditional logistic regression** should be used, as an extension to the **McNemar's test** for paired (non-**independent**) proportions. **Polytomous logistic regression** and **ordered logistic regression** are used for **nominal** and **ordinal** outcomes. An example of a logistic regression analysis is given in Box 11.

Lognormal distribution

Positively **skewed** distribution whose log values display a **normal distribution**.

Mann–Whitney U-test

Significance test for comparing the distribution of a given variable between two groups. The test is a **non-parametric** alternative to the independent samples **t-test**. It is used when the data are **ordinal** or when the requirement

BOX 11
Silfverdal S *et al.* (1997). Protective effect of breastfeeding on invasive haemophilus influenzae (HI) infection: a case-control study in Swedish preschool children. *Int J Epidemiol* **26**: 443–450.
Prospective case-control study carried out over a period of 6 years, from 1987 to 1992 (before introduction of general Hib vaccination in Sweden). Fifty-four cases with invasive HI infection and 139 matched controls were assembled over the study period. The risk factors investigated were: day-care outside of the home, short duration of breastfeeding (<13 weeks), passive smoking, low socioeconomic level of the household, many siblings, allergy, frequent infections, repeated antibiotic treatments and immunoglobin deficiency. The results of multiple logistic regression analysis showed two variables to have a significant association with HI infection:

Predictor variables	OR	95% CI
1 Short duration of breastfeeding	3.79	1.6 to 8.8
2 History of frequent infections	4.49	1.0 to 21.0

Interpretation:
Although very imprecise, these results suggest a protective effect of breastfeeding against HI infection ('risk' decreased by a factor of 3.79, which could be as low as 1.6 or as high as 8.8), and an increased risk of infection with frequent general infections ('risk' increased by a factor of 4.49, which could be as low as 1, no effect, or as high as 21!).

for **normality** is not met. For **paired data**, the **Wilcoxon matched pairs signed rank test** should be used. These tests are based on **ranks** (ordering of the data) and not on the actual values. The Wilcoxon rank sum T-test for independent samples is an equivalent to the Mann–Whitney U-test.

MANOVA **Multivariate** equivalent to **analysis of variance (ANOVA)**. Commonly used in psychological research. It is used to test for group differences in profile of measurements, as opposed to the use of ANOVA to test for group differences in single measurements. MANOVA provides the **significance test** for linear **discriminant analysis**.

Mantel–Haenszel χ^2 test **Significance test** for comparing **proportions** or **odds** in the presence of **confounding** factors. For example, we may be interested in the risk (proportion) of cervical cancer in women taking the contraceptive pill for 10 years or more, compared to those who have taken it for less than 10 years. Age is related to the risk of cervical cancer. Also, older women are more likely to have been on the pill for longer. It is therefore necessary to separate the effects of the contraceptive pill on cervical cancer from the effects of age. After **stratification** by categories of the confounding variable – age, results in each **stratum** are pooled together to produce a single summary test across all *strata*. The number of **degrees of freedom** for this test is always one.

Mantel–Haenszel estimates	Method which combines the **relative risk estimates** of several **two-by-two tables** to produce a single summary, which is a weighted average across the individual tables. The analysis of **case-control studies** and **meta-analysis** are common applications of the method. Weights are usually directly proportional to the degree of certainty or **precision (2)** of the individual estimates (or inversely proportional to the their **variance**). Thus, larger studies are usually given more weight than smaller ones.
Masking	See **blinding**.
Matching	Selection of **controls** in **case-control studies,** with the view to ensure a similar distribution of important **risk** and/or **prognostic factors** (frequently age and sex) in the two study groups (cases and controls). Matching can be (a) individual or pairwise, or (b) by **stratum**, group or frequency matching. In the latter, an equal distribution of prognostic factors is achieved by ensuring that cases and controls have, overall, similar numbers of subjects with the same characteristics, for the relevant prognostic factors (e.g. similar proportion of males, or of people over 65 years). As with **paired proportions**, the **McNemar's test** and **conditional logistic regression** are appropriate for the analysis of individually matched designs. The **chi-squared test, Mantel–Haenszel estimates**, the **Mantel–Haenszel chi-squared test** and **logistic regression** are indicated in stratum matching. When matching, it is important to be aware of the risk of **overmatching**.
Maximum likelihood	Alternative method of fitting **regression models**. Especially indicated for **Cox, logistic** and **Poisson regression**, where the **least squares** method is not appropriate. [The term likelihood measures the probability of a body of data given that certain values are chosen as the model's parameters (CLAYTON and HILLS, 1993). The values which maximize this probability are said to produce the maximum likelihood model for the data.]
McNemar's test	**Significance test** which is a special form of the **chi-squared test** used in the analysis of **paired proportions**. See Appendix C for a worked example.

Mean   Measure of the centre of a **distribution**. The mean is a reliable measure of centre or 'average' if the variable being summarized has a symmetrical distribution. If this is not the case, the arithmetic mean does not provide a fair summary for the bulk of the data, since it is influenced by extreme observations or **outliers** (Figure 5, p 27). The formula for calculating the mean is:

$$\bar{x} = \frac{\text{sum of individual observations}}{\text{sample size}} = \frac{\Sigma x_i}{n}$$

The **standard deviation** is commonly used to express the spread of individual observations around the mean.

Median   Measure of the centre of a **distribution**. As opposed to the **mean**, it is said to be a **robust** measure, given that it is not greatly affected by the presence of **outliers** (Figure 7, p 27). When the data are sorted according to increasing values of the variable of interest, the median is the middle value, i.e. the value which divides the data in half: 50% of observations have values lower than the median and 50% have values greater than the median (Figure 4, p 8). If the total number of observations is an even number, the median is then the average of the two central values. The median is also referred to as the 50th **percentile**. It should be computed when the mean is inappropriate (e.g. **skewed** distributions). When the median is used, the spread of the observations can be expressed by the relevant percentiles, and commonly by the **interquartile range (IQR)**.

Meta-analysis   Statistical analysis which combines the results of the individual studies used in a **systematic review**, producing a quantitative summary across the different studies. It uses methods such as **Mantel–Haenszel estimates** and **Peto's method** to calculate these summaries. Meta-analysis has the virtue of increasing the **sample size** available to **estimate**, say, the benefits of a given treatment. The technique is commonly used for **randomized controlled trials** of therapies or interventions. However, it can also be used for studies on **risk factors** or **diagnostic tests**, for example. Issues around meta-analysis are **publication bias**, **heterogeneity** (which also involves decisions on the use of **fixed** or **random effects** models), use of individual data from all studies involved (if obtainable) or aggregated data, i.e. estimates such as **odds ratios** computed in each individual study (commonly used), to cite a few. Readers are referred to CHALMERS and ALTMAN (eds, 1995) for a full discussion. Figure 9 shows a typical meta-analysis graph (SMITH *et al.*, 1993, Figure 2), in which the results from individual studies are displayed on either side of a vertical line which represents absence of treatment effect. This allows the magnitude and direction of treatment effect in each study to be assessed. In addition, **confidence intervals** are also presented, which can readily give information on the **statistical significance** and **precision (2)** of the individual estimates. See also **cumulative meta-analysis**.

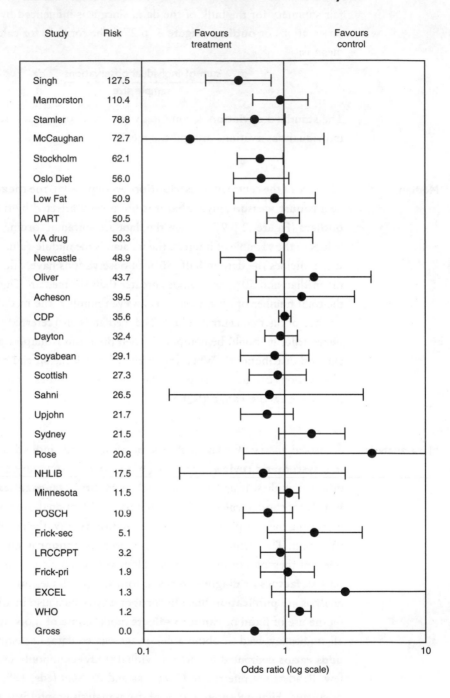

Figure 9 Meta-analysis of the effect of cholestrol lowering on total mortality, in relation to risk of death from coronary heart disease per 1000 PYAR [reproduced with permission from Smith, Song and Sheldon (1993). *Br Med J* **306**: 1367–1373].

Minimization   Quasi-**random** method of allocating patients to the different treatments in a **clinical trial**. The rationale behind minimization is the need to produce treatment groups which have similar distributions for important **prognostic factors**. The method is useful especially when dealing with small size trials, where simple **randomization** often produces unbalanced groups. See Pocock (1983) for a worked example.

Model   In the context of **regression** analysis, a model is an equation which summarizes the relationship between an **outcome variable** and one or more **predictor variables**. When there is a single predictor variable the general form of the equation is:

Predicted outcome $= \hat{y}$

$= a + bx$

$=$ constant value $+$ (rate of change in y per unit of x) $\times$ (value of x)

where $\hat{y}$ (read 'y hat') is the predicted value of the outcome variable, x is the value of the predictor variable, a is the **intercept** and b is the **regression coefficient** (Box 12). The difference between observed and **predicted** values is the **residual**. **Multiple regression** models are developed to allow for more than one predictor variable.

BOX 12
From **Figure 15**, p 67.
The equation that summarizes the relationship between bone density (study units) and age (in years) in postmenopausal women (random sample of 100 women) can be written as:
Bone density = 62.7 − 0.47 × age

Interpretation:		
1 Negative relationship: regression coefficient for age has negative sign. On average, a 4.7 decrease for each ten year age increase.		
2 Intercept or base value for bone density: 62.7.		
3 Other quantities of interest:		
P-value	<0.00005	predictor variable (age) statistically significant (association not likely to be due to chance).
R-squared	= 0.17	approximately 17% of the variability in bone density can be explained by age.
Adj R-squared	= 0.16	
Root mean square error (MSE)	= 6.07	
		average prediction error.

Multiple regression

Process of fitting a **regression model** with more than one **predictor variable**, as opposed to **simple regression** analysis. In particular, multiple regression is used in cases where it is necessary to adjust for **confounders** or check for the presence of **interactions**. The general form of the equation is:

$$\hat{y} = a + b_1x_1 + b_2x_2 + b_3x_3 + \ldots$$

where $\hat{y}$ (read 'y hat') is the predicted value for the **outcome variable**, x_1, x_2, x_3, ... are the values of the predictor variables, b_1, b_2, b_3, ... are the **regression coefficients** and a is the **intercept** or constant. Each predictor is now associated with a regression coefficient defining its relationship with the outcome variable (Box 2, p 3).

Multiple significance testing

Multiple **significance tests** which are carried out on the same body of data. An example of this is **sub-group analysis** where first an overall test is performed, and then, subsequent tests are carried out for sub-groups of subjects sharing similar characteristics. For example, in the ISIS-2 trial (Box 1, p 1) comparing aspirin versus **placebo** for the treatment of acute myocardial infarction, one may be interested in making this comparison within different age groups, since aspirin could be effective if used say, in younger patients, but not in older patients. If three age groups are defined, three statistical tests will be performed, the likelihood of a **type I error** increasing with the number of tests carried out. Two approaches to dealing with this problem are the use of corrections (e.g. **Bonferroni** or **Dunnett's**) or the adoption of a more stringent cut-off point for acceptance of **statistical significance** (e.g. 0.01 instead of the conventional 0.05). Ideally, such analyses should be planned *a priori* to avoid spurious findings.

Multistage sampling

Sampling method where the selection of study units is done in more than one stage, going from the larger to the smaller units in a **population**. For example, in two-stage sampling, a **random sample** of general practices in a given area may be taken in the first stage (first-stage units) and patients, second-stage units, subsequently chosen (also at random) from the selected practices. The method should be performed with 'proportional probability to size' with replacement, if the first-stage units have different sizes, in order to give second-stage units the same probability of being selected. Multistage sampling differs from **cluster sampling**, in which all second-stage units within the first-stage units sampled are selected.

Multivariate methods

Term frequently used to refer to statistical methods employed in any analysis involving more than one **predictor variable**, such as **multiple regression** and **logistic regression**. In the strict sense, it refers to methods for analysing two or more **outcome variables** simultaneously. Methods commonly used are **cluster analysis, discriminant analysis, factor analysis, MANOVA** and **principal components analysis**. The analysis of **repeated measurements** can be seen as a special application of multivariate methods.

N-of-I trials

Clinical trials conducted by clinicians on individual patients, in the absence of other evidence on which to substantiate the choice of treatments or other clinical actions for the same patients. Ethical considerations and patient collaboration are important, as they should be in any medical investigation. N-of-1 trials are for obvious reasons more limited than larger clinical trials, but can still be useful if conducted scientifically. This involves **controlling, randomization** and **blind** assessment of responses, and also repetition of observation. SACKETT *et al.* (1991, 1997) recommend the use of pairs of two periods, in which the treatment in question and a **placebo** or an alternative treatment are both administered in random order. These two-period pairs are repeated until evidence of benefit or lack of benefit emerges. N-of-1 trials are in many ways similar to **crossover trials**, not only in that patients are their own controls, but also because they raise the same practical issues.

Negative predictive value

See **predictive values**.

Nominal variable

Categorical variable whose categories are not ordered (e.g. eye colour, nationality, blood group).

Non-parametric methods

Statistical methods for the analysis of data which do not conform with the requirements for **parametric methods**. Common non-parametric tests are the **Mann–Whitney U-test**, the **Wilcoxon matched pairs signed rank test**, the **Kruskal–Wallis test** and **rank correlation** (Figure 18, p 77). **Interquartile ranges** (Figure 4, p 8) are an example of a non-parametric descriptive measure. These methods are based on the **ranks** given to the values of the observations, rather than the actual observations. Data **transformations** (for example, to a logarithmic scale) may be an alternative to using non-parametric methods.

Normal distribution

or Gaussian distribution. Theoretical **distribution** which has the form of a bell-shaped curve and is perfectly symmetrical about its centre. Figure 10 shows the **histogram** of a variable with an approximately normal distribution, and the shape of the corresponding theoretical normal curve. The normal distribution is totally defined by two parameters: the **mean**, reflecting its centre, and the **standard deviation (SD)**, reflecting the spread of individual observations. Biological and other measurements frequently follow an approximate (or empirical) normal distribution. Because of the mathematical properties of the normal curve, we can calculate the probability of obtaining a measurement above or below any given value, provided the variable in question follows an approximate normal distribution (e.g. height). Tables of the normal distribution give these probabilities for the 'standard normal distribution' (i.e. a normal distribution with mean 0 and standard deviation 1). For normal distributions with other values for the mean and standard deviation, the above probabilities can be obtained by converting the original observations into **z-scores** (values expressed in units of SD). Since many statistical methods (**parametric methods**) are based on the properties and/or **assumption** of a normal distribution, this is a desirable property for **quantitative variables**.

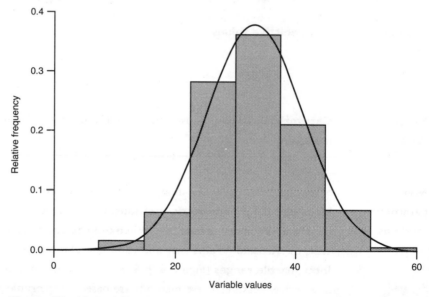

Figure 10 Normal distribution.

Normal plot

Graphical display of a **quantitative variable**, used to visually assess the **assumption** of **normality**. Figures 11 and 12 below show examples of a normal plot for a variable which is normally distributed (same as in Figure 10), and for a variable displaying a positive **skew** – with greater frequency of lower values than higher values (Figure 17, p 76). The vertical

(y) axis represents the values of the variable in the original scale, and the horizontal (x) axis gives the inverse normal for the same variable (i.e. it assumes the variable follows a perfect normal distribution, given its **mean** and **standard deviation**). If the variable in question has a normal (or approximately normal) distribution, the plot results in a fairly straight line. A concave curve is produced for variables with a positive skew, and a convex curve for variables presenting a negative skew. A more formal way of assessing normality is by the Wilk or **Shapiro–Wilk test**.

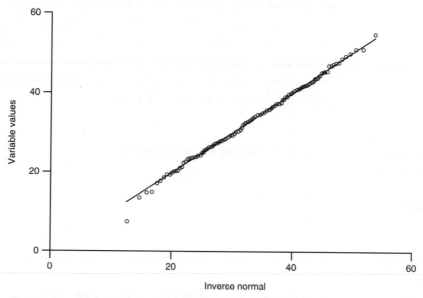

Figure 11 Normal plot: normally distributed variable.

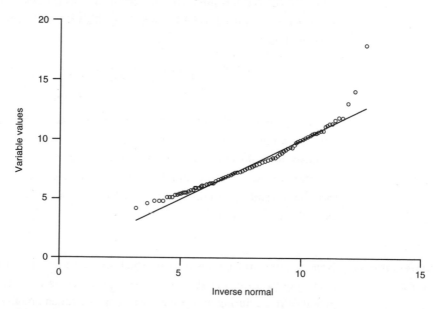

Figure 12 Normal plot: positively skewed variable.

Null hypothesis (H$_0$ or NH)	Hypothesis put forward when carrying out **significance tests**, which states: (a) there are no differences between groups being compared (e.g. aspirin and **placebo** equally effective in preventing death in patients with acute myocardial infarction), or (b) there is no relationship or association between variables (e.g. caloric intake and body mass index), in the relevant **populations** (i.e. all people similar to those participating in a study). Significance tests are carried out on the assumption that H$_0$ is true. It is then necessary to decide the deviation of the data obtained from what would be expected if H$_0$ were true. This is expressed as a probability or **P-value**. The smaller the *P*-value, the lower the likelihood of obtaining the result observed in the study **sample** (or a more extreme one) if H$_0$ is in fact true. In these cases, differences and associations observed are declared **statistically significant**, i.e. unlikely to be due to chance, and H$_0$ is rejected. If *P*-values are large, conventionally >0.05, there is not sufficient evidence to reject the NH (*not the same as 'accepting' the NH!*).
Number needed to harm (NNH)	See **number needed to treat (NNT)**.
Number needed to treat (NNT)	Measure of the impact of a treatment or intervention. It states how many patients need to be treated with the treatment in question, in order to prevent an event which would otherwise occur. The **risk** of the event in question in patients given the new intervention, and in patients given standard treatment (or no treatment) need to be known. From Table 1 (p 15), the NNT is calculated as:

$$\text{NNT} = \frac{1}{\text{risk}_2 - \text{risk}_1} = \frac{1}{\text{ARD}} = \frac{1}{\dfrac{b}{b+d} - \dfrac{a}{a+c}}$$

	where risk$_2$ is the risk in the control group and risk$_1$ is the risk in the intervention group (both expressed as proportions). Because it is based on the **absolute difference in risks (ARD)**, it is possible for a treatment of only moderate or little efficacy (in relative terms) to have a small NNT, and therefore considerable impact when used to treat a common disease. An example is given in Box 13.
Observational study	Non-experimental investigation in which subjects are not submitted to actual interventions. Instead, subjects can be kept under observation for a given period of time, during which measurements are taken and events registered, or they can be interviewed and/or examined at a particular point in time.

BOX 13
From **Box 1**, p 1.
The NNT is calculated as 1/ARD (i.e. if 2.4 deaths are prevented per 100 patients treated, how many patients are necessary to prevent 1 death?). The calculation gives:
NNT = 1/0.24 = 42
This shows the intervention (aspirin here) to have considerable impact on vascular mortality in patients with AMI. If aspirin has any serious side-effects, the 'number needed to harm' should also be computed, and the two results, NNT and NNH, considered when making clinical and policy decisions.

Examples of this type of study are **cross-sectional, cohort** and **case-control** studies. ROTHMAN (1986) gives a full discussion of issues related to observational studies. For an overview see WALD (1996).

Odds
Ratio of the number of times an event occurs to the number of times it does not occur, out of a given number of chances (Box 4, p 14). Odds are used to convey the idea of '**risk**' although the two are only approximately the same when considering rare events (e.g. winning the lottery). For a common event, such as a newborn baby being a boy or a girl, the probability or risk is roughly 0.5 or 50%, but the odds are 1 (50:50).

Odds ratio (OR)
Ratio of two **odds**, often used in epidemiological studies (in particular **case-control studies**) or **clinical trials** as a measure of **relative risk**, to compare **exposed** vs non-exposed or intervention vs **control** groups (Box 4, p 14). If the odds are the same in the two groups their ratio will be 1. From Table 1 (p 15):

$$OR = \frac{\text{odds in exposed}}{\text{odds in non-exposed}} = \frac{a}{b} \div \frac{c}{d} = \frac{ad}{bc}$$

For rare diseases the OR and the **risk ratio** (calculated using the actual **risks**, not the odds) will be very similar. Box 14 gives a table for converting ORs into a useful measure of impact, the **number needed to treat (NNT)**.

One-sided test
Significance test which only explores one alternative hypothesis to the **null hypothesis (NH)**, when comparisons are being made. For example, if comparing the **risk** of disease experienced by the intervention and **placebo** groups in a **clinical trial**, the NH states that the risk of disease is the same in

<table>
<tr><td colspan="11" align="center">**BOX 14**</td></tr>
</table>

Sackett D, Richardson W, Rosenberg W, Haynes R (1997). *Evidence-based medicine; how to practice and teach EBM.* Churchill Livingstone (reproduced with permission).

Translating ORs to NNTs:

Because results from clinical trials and meta-analyses are often presented as ORs, the table below can be used to convert these into a measure of treatment impact, the number needed to treat (NNT). Another quantity, the **patient expected event rate (PEER)**, is also needed for using the table.

		Odds ratios (OR)								
		0.90	0.85	0.80	0.75	0.70	0.65	0.60	0.55	0.5
Your	0.05	209	139	104	83	69	59	52	46	41
patient's	0.10	110	73	54	43	36	31	27	24	21
expected	0.20	61	40	30	24	20	17	14	13	11
event	0.30	46	30	22	18	14	12	10	9	8
rate	0.40	40	26	19	15	12	10	9	8	7
(PEER)	0.50	38	25	18	14	11	9	8	7	6
	0.70	44	28	20	16	13	10	9	7	6
	0.90	101	64	46	34	27	22	18	15	12

The numbers in the body of the table are the NNTs for the corresponding odds ratios at that particular patient's expected event rate (PEER).

To calculate the NNT for any OR and PEER:

$$NNT = \frac{1 - [PEER \times (1 - OR)]}{(1 - PEER) \times PEER \times (1 - OR)}$$

the two groups. In a one-sided test, as opposed to a **two-sided test**, the alternative hypothesis tested is that the risk in the intervention group is *less* than the risk in the **control** group. The possibility that the risk in the intervention group could be *greater* than in the control group is disregarded. A one-sided test should never be used unless there is absolute certainty only one alternative to the NH is possible. An example is given in Box 15.

One-way ANOVA

Analysis of variance of data classified according to a single factor or characteristic. For example, one may wish to compare the mean birthweight among different ethnic groups (classifying factor). As with the **independent** samples **t-test**, the **assumptions** of **normality of distributions** and similar **variances** in the groups being compared are required. The **null hypothesis** of no difference between the groups is tested by the **F-test**.

+--+
| **BOX 15** |
+--+
| Roberts M *et al.* (1984). The Edinburgh randomized trial of screening for breast |
| cancer: description of method. *Br J Cancer* **50**: 1–6. |
+--+
| The UK seven-year trial of breast cancer screening started in 1979. Edinburgh |
| was one of the participating centres, with 65 000 women aged 45 to 65 years |
| enrolled, in clusters defined by their general practices. The researchers in this |
| trial based the sample size calculations on the assumption that the outcome for |
| women screened could not be worst than for women not screened. Although |
| this seems reasonable, there are well-known harmful effects of screening that |
| should not be overlooked in an investigation of this type. |
+--+

Ordered logistic regression

Logistic regression which is used when the **outcome variable** is an **ordinal variable** (e.g. severity of pain, categorized as no pain, minimal pain, moderate pain and severe pain).

Ordinal variable

Categorical variable in which the different levels of the variable are ordered. Going through successive levels represents successive 'increases' or 'decreases' in the characteristic conveyed by the variable. An example of an ordinal variable is 'severity of pain': no pain, minimal pain, moderate pain, severe pain. Unlike **interval** or **ratio variables**, the differences between any two consecutive levels of an ordinal variable do not necessarily represent increments of the same magnitude. For example, the difference between no pain and minimal pain is unlikely to be the same as between minimal pain and moderate pain. Nonetheless, it is important to analyse this type of data with special methods (e.g. chi-squared test for **trend, Kruskal–Wallis test**) and not with methods used for **nominal variables**.

Outcome variable

also dependent or response variable. It represents the characteristic or measurement (e.g. death or cholesterol levels) which is used to test the main hypothesis in an investigation. In the context of **regression** it is usually called the **y-variable**, and represents the observed values of y. The **predicted** values of y ($\hat{y}$ – read 'y hat') are those obtained by any given regression **model**.

Outliers

Values in a set of observations, which are much higher or lower than the 'average'. An important consequence of the presence of outliers is that data will not be **normally distributed**. Thus, when comparing groups using a **t-test** or when constructing a **reference range**, for example, it may be necessary to **transform** the data or use **non-parametric methods**. In the context of **regression** and **correlation**, outliers tend to dominate and affect

measures of association between two variables, as expressed by the
regression coefficient (and **intercept**), and the **correlation coefficient**.
However, outlying observations should never be discarded without careful
consideration. The identification of outliers is important and can be done by
simple graphical methods. Figure 13 shows the graphical display of a
regression analysis. The solid regression line was estimated without taking
the outlying observations into account. The effect of these outliers on the
regression line would be as follows:

1 Outlier in *y*. Intercept: slightly increased; slope: slightly decreased; its
   own **residual** (vertical distance to solid line): moderate size.
2 Outlier in *x*. Intercept: moderately increased; slope: moderately
   decreased; its own residual: small size.
3 Outlier in *y* and *x*. Intercept: greatly increased; slope: negative (direction
   of relationship is inverted); its own residual: small or very small size.
   Outlier 3 is an influential observation.

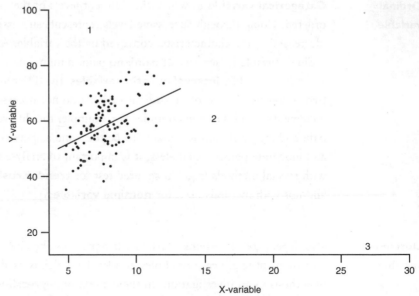

Figure 13 Regression line with three outliers.

**Over-
matching**

In the context of **matching**, occurs when cases and **controls** are matched for
variables which are *not* **confounding** factors. For example, if cases and
controls are matched for parental alcohol consumption in a **case-control
study** investigating the relationship between parental smoking and asthma in
children, cases and controls will be 'made' to have similar smoking
exposures since smoking is frequently associated with alcohol consumption.
However, asthma in children is not related to parental drinking habits (at
least not directly!), and, as a result, it may be wrongly concluded that
parental smoking and asthma in children are not related.

Overview See **systematic review**.

P-value In the context of **significance tests**, the *P*-value represents the probability that a given difference (or a difference more extreme) is observed in a study **sample** (between **means**, **proportions**, etc.), when in reality such a difference does not exist in the relevant **population** (all individuals similar to those in the study sample). Small *P*-values indicate stronger evidence to reject the **null hypothesis (NH)** of no difference. For example, a *P*-value = 0.004 can be interpreted as a 4 in 1000 chance of observing a difference of a given magnitude (or a more extreme one), say between two means, when, in the population (i.e. if we could have carried out a study with *all* similar patients), the two groups being compared have similar means. Conventionally, a difference is said to be **statistically significant** if the corresponding *P*-value is ≤ 0.05. However, it is preferable to report exact *P*-values rather than the usual 'NS' (non-significant) or '*P* < 0.05': it is clear that the difference between *P* = 0.049 and *P* = 0.051 is too small to deserve such dichotomy. When looking at **correlation** or **regression**, the NH being tested is that the correlation or regression **coefficients** are equal to 0 (no relationship between the variables in question). The *P*-value may also be thought of as the probability that a **type I error** has occurred. See Box 16 for an example from the ISIS-2 study.

BOX 16
From **Box 1**, p 1.
The probability that an absolute risk difference (ARD) of 2.4% or greater could have been found in a study of this size, when, in fact, it is simply a chance finding, is less than 1 in 100 000 (*P* < 0.00001). The results of the comparison of aspirin vs no aspirin (with respect to 5-week vascular mortality) are therefore statistically significant.

Paired data See **independence**.

Paired t-test Special form of the **t-test** which is used to compare the **means** of two paired variables (i.e. not **independent**). A common example of paired data are measurements taken in the same group of subjects *before* and *after* some treatment or intervention. The number of **degrees of freedom (df)** for the paired *t*-test is $n - 1$, where *n* is the number of pairs. An **assumption** of the paired *t*-test is that the *differences* (for example, 'after'− 'before' difference) are **normally distributed**. The **Wilcoxon test for matched pairs** can be used as an alternative or with paired **ordinal** data. See Appendix C for a worked example.

Parallel design	Study design used in **clinical trials**. As opposed to **crossover designs** where subjects act as their own **control**, in a parallel design two (or more) separate groups of subjects each receive just one of the treatments being compared, one of them acting as the control group.
Parametric methods	Statistical methods of data analysis which rely on one or more distributional **assumptions** for the data being analysed, commonly **normality** (data follow an approximate normal distribution) and **homoscedasticity** (i.e. constant **variability**). Examples are **t-tests** (for comparing means) and **Pearson's correlation**.
Patient expected event rate (PEER)	Estimate of a particular patient's risk of disease over a period of time (obtained from research). The PEER can be used in conjunction with the **RRR (relative risk reduction)** estimate from a study to give a particularized **absolute risk difference (ARD)**, which can be used to calculate the **NNT (number needed to treat)** for the same patient. Box 17 gives a nomogram to convert PEERs into NNTs, using RRRs.
Pearson's correlation coefficient (r)	or product-moment correlation coefficient. Measure of the strength of the *linear* relationship between two **quantitative variables**. r can take any value between -1 and $+1$, where $r = -1$ represents a perfect negative correlation, $r = +1$ a perfect positive correlation, and $r = 0$ no linear relationship. Thus, the absolute value of r indicates the strength of the linear relationship and its sign the direction of the relationship. It should be noted that $r = 0$ does not imply no relationship at all, but the absence of a *linear* one. Another way of assessing the strength of a relationship is to compute the square of r, i.e. **r-squared (r^2)**. The **statistical significance** of the correlation coefficient can be assessed by computing an associated **P-value**. It should be noted that the latter cannot give any information on the strength of the relationship itself: a small P-value is not synonymous with strong association. An **assumption** of **parametric** correlation is that one or both variables (for significance testing or confidence intervals) are **normally distributed**, due to the effect **outliers** (i.e. extreme observations) may have on r. When required assumptions cannot be met, **rank correlation** can be used instead. Figure 14 shows a **scatterplot** of the association between bone density (study units) and age (in years), in postmenopausal women, from the example in Box 12.
Percentiles	For a given variable with values sorted in ascending order, percentiles (or quantiles) are the values of the variable below which a certain percentage of the observations is found. Thus, for a given set of measurements, 10% of the

---

BOX 17

Sackett D, Richardson W, Rosenberg W, Haynes R (1997). *Evidence-based medicine; how to practice and teach EBM.* Churchill Livingstone (reproduced with permission).

Translating PEERs and RRRs into NNTs:

To use the nomogram, a straight line is drawn through the value of the patient's PEER and study RRR, and the resulting NNT can be read off.

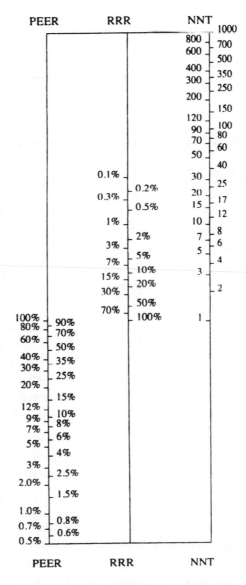

Reprinted with permission from Chatelier G *et al.* (1996). The number to treat: a clinically useful nomogram in its proper context. *Br Med J* **312**: 426–429.

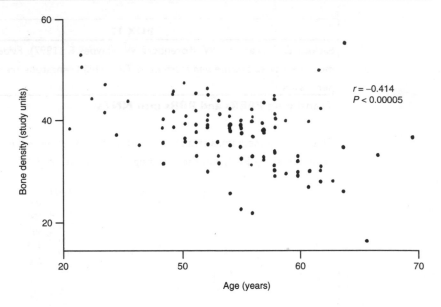

Figure 14 Scatterplot of bone density vs age: negative correlation.

observations have values below the value corresponding to the 10th percentile. Special percentiles are the **median** (50th percentile), and the 25th and 75th percentiles, also known as **quartiles**. The following numbers are height measurements (in feet) for a group of 13 people. The percentiles of this distribution are shown in the row below the measurements:

<5.2 5.2 5.3 5.3 5.4 5.4 5.5 5.6 5.6 5.7 5.8 5.9 6.1>
<   10th   25th   50th   75th   90th   >

Period effect   In the context of **crossover trials**, it refers to the effect of time on disease, as measured by relevant **outcomes**. This acknowledges the fact that disease, and therefore patients' responses, may vary from one period to the next, regardless of any concomitant treatments. This is sometimes due to learning effects (for example, learning to cope with pain). The presence of a period effect is not as serious as the presence of a **treatment-period interaction**, since treatment order is **randomly** allocated in crossover trials. Thus, a simple period effect should affect all study treatments equally.

Person-time at risk   Sum of the individual lengths of time each subject is under observation in a **follow-up study** (**observational study** or **clinical trial**). It can be estimated as the number at risk of the event of interest (contracting a disease or dying) multiplied by the average length of the study period. Usually, time is expressed in years – person-years at risk (PYAR) – but it can also be expressed in days, weeks, etc. Person-time at risk is the denominator in the computation of **rates**. Box 18 gives a worked example of PYAR calculations.

BOX 18

Worked example:

Follow-up study with five subjects (not really a good idea!). Two deaths (event of interest) are observed during the follow-up period. The length of follow-up for each subject is:

Subject	Duration of follow-up	
1	3 years	**PYAR =**
2	2 years and 7 months	12 years and 4 months
3	1 year and 9 months	= 12.333 years
4	3 years	**Mortality rate** = 2 per 12.333 PYAR
5	2 years	= 0.16 per PYAR = 16 per 100 PYAR

Interpretation:

If a person, with similar characteristics to the above cohort, is followed up for one year, the 'risk' of dying is 0.16. In other words, over 100 years of observation (e.g. 50 people followed up for 2 years each) 16 deaths are expected to occur.

Peto's method	Statistical method of combining **odds ratios (OR)** in a **meta-analysis**. The method is particularly indicated for **clinical trials**, where the **sample sizes** of the groups being compared tend to be fairly similar. It can lead to **biased** results if the estimated OR is far from 1. Peto's method is based on the ratio of observed to **expected frequencies**, obtained with the results displayed in a **two-by-two table** (these are the frequencies for cell *a* in Table 1, p 15 – treatment YES/outcome YES). **Mantel–Haenszel estimates** are an alternative way of combining results in meta-analyses.
Placebo	Inactive or dummy treatment which, in a **clinical trial**, is given to the **control** group in order to prevent **information biases**, since it enables both patients and researchers to remain **blind** to the treatments given. Placebos must be similar to active treatments (colour, taste, mode of administration), if they are going to have the desired effect.
Poisson regression	**Regression** method for the analysis of counts (e.g. number of cases of a rare disease in different geographical areas) and **rates** (e.g. mortality rates).
Polytomous logistic regression	**Logistic regression** method which is used when the **categorical outcome** has more than two unordered categories (e.g. different conditions associated

with chest pain – angina, acute myocardial infarction, acid reflux, pneumonia, etc., or different categories of cause of death). Also termed multinomial logistic regression.

Population

See **target population**.

Population attributable risk

Measure of the impact an **exposure** or **risk factor** has on a given **population**, in terms of excess risk of disease. It depends not only on how strongly the exposure in question is associated with a particular disease, but, more importantly, on the **prevalence** of the exposure. It is calculated as follows:

Population attributable risk =

incidence in population − incidence in non-exposed

As with the **attributable risk**, the population attributable risk can be expressed as a fraction of the population's **incidence** of disease, the population proportional attributable risk or attributable fraction (PAF):

Population proportional attributable risk =
$$\frac{\text{incidence in population} - \text{incidence in non-exposed}}{\text{incidence in population}}$$

The example given in Box 19 (WALD, 1996) illustrates the above concepts.

Positive predictive value

See **predictive values**.

Posttest probability

In the context of **diagnostic testing**, it is an individual's probability of actually having a given condition, given a particular test result. It depends not only on the **prevalence** of the condition in question, but also on the **likelihood ratio (LR)** for that test result. It is calculated as follows:

$$\text{Posttest probability} = \frac{\text{posttest odds}}{\text{posttest odds} + 1}$$

where posttest odds = LR × pretest odds (see **pretest probability**). The posttest probability of disease given a particular test result is also known as the **predictive value** of the same result. See SACKETT *et al.* (1991) for further discussion. Box 20 shows an example of these calculations with a diagnostic tool for alcohol abuse.

BOX 19

Doll R, Peto R et al. (1994). Mortality in relation to smoking: 40 years' observations on male British doctors. Br Med J **309**: 901–911.

This study has become a classic example to demonstrate the ideas of relative and absolute effect. It considers the association between smoking and mortality to lung cancer and ischaemic heart disease. In the first case, the association is rather strong (RR = 14.9) and in the second case, it is weak (RR = 1.6). However, the impact of the exposure (cigarette smoking) is greater for ischaemic heart disease than for lung cancer (as judged by the absolute excess risk), due to the fact that the former is more common and has a higher mortality rate than the latter.

Cause of death	Age standardized annual death rate per 100 000			Absolute excess risk (per 100 000 per year)
	non-smokers	current smokers	RR	
Lung cancer	14	209	14.9	195
Ischaemic heart disease	572	892	1.6	320

WALD gives a hypothetical but realistic example of how the above RRs and ARDs could be translated into number of premature deaths prevented in a particular population, with a given prevalence of exposure to cigarette smoking. It assumes approximately 30% of men in the age group 45–54 (the population) to be smokers, and the risk of dying from ischaemic heart disease to be 3 per 1000 per year among smokers and 1 per 1000 per year among non-smokers (RR = 3). The PAF can be calculated using this equivalent formula:

$$\text{PAF} = \frac{p(\text{RR} - 1)}{p(\text{RR} - 1) + 1} = \frac{0.3(3 - 1)}{0.3(3 - 1) + 1} = \frac{0.6}{1.6} = 38\%$$

Interpretation:
38% of IHD deaths in this population of 45 to 54-year-old males can be attributed to smoking, i.e. prevented (in principle) by removal of the exposure.

Power

Probability of finding a difference, in a research study, to be **statistically significant**, when this difference actually exists. For example, 80% power in a **clinical trial** of size N, represents an 80% chance of detecting a given difference say, between two proportions – equal to some prespecified value, which is termed 'smallest **clinically significant** difference' – with a small associated **P-value**. The power of a particular study is increased by increasing its **sample size**. In addition, with **quantitative outcomes**, the greater the **variability** of the individual measurements, the lower the power of the study. The level of significance required for the results (P-value or **type I error**) also determines the power of a study. The complement of power is the **type II error (β)** (power = $1 - \beta$). ALTMAN (1991) gives a nomogram for

BOX 20			
Sackett *et al.* (1991). *Clinical Epidemiology: A Basic Science for Clinical Medicine.* Little, Brown & Co.			
The CAGE questionnaire for alcohol abuse:			
C Ever CUT down on drinking?			
A Do people ever ANNOY you about your drinking?			
G Ever feel GUILTY?			
E Ever need an EYE-OPENER?			
CAGE results			
No. of Yes answers	**Abusers**	**Non-abusers**	**LR**
3 or 4	60	1	60/117 ÷1/401 = 250
2	28	14	28/117÷14/401 = 7
1	11	28	11/117÷28/401 = 1.3
0	18	358	18/117÷358/401=0.2
	117	401	

1 If we believe a given patient has 50% chance of being an alcohol abuser, the pre-test odds are:

$$\{\text{pre-test probability}/(1 - \text{pre-test probability})\} = 1.$$

2 If the patient responds 'yes' to two questions, LR = 7 and post-test odds = 7 also (1×7).

3 This corresponds to a post-test probability of 87.5%:

$$\{\text{post-test odds}/(\text{post-test odds} + 1)\}.$$

power calculations (Box 21). KIRKWOOD (1988) gives formulae for a number of **summary measures,** for both power and **precision (2)** calculations. CLINSTAT (BLAND, 1991) carries out a number of power calculations.

Precision (1)   Number of significant digits obtained for a measurement. For example, the height of an individual recorded as 1.734 m is more precise than if recorded as 1.7 m. It is important to note that a precise measurement is not necessarily an **accurate** or correct one. When reporting results from research, care should be taken to avoid spurious (i.e. unnecessary) precision.

Precision (2)   In the context of **estimation,** this term refers to the magnitude of the **standard error (SE)** of an estimate. This is reflected in the width of the **confidence interval (CI)** constructed around the same estimate. Wide CIs reflect considerable uncertainty about the true **population** values, and stem from small **sample sizes** and/or large **variability** of measurements. A precise estimate is only useful if it is also **unbiased.**

BOX 21

Altman D (1991). *Practical statistics for medical research*. Chapman & Hall (reproduced with permission).

Nomogram for power calculations:

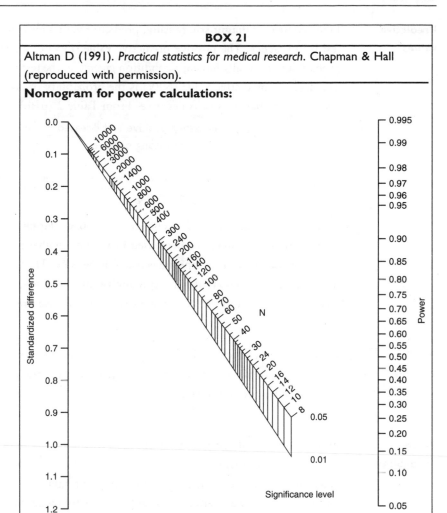

Reproduced with permission from Altman D (1982). How large a sample? In *Statistics in Practice* (eds S Gore and D Altman), p 7, Figure 2. British Medical Association.

To use this nomogram, differences are standardized, by dividing the smallest clinically significant difference by the **standard deviation** of the measurements (for numerical data), or by $\sqrt{[p(1-p)]}$, where p is the average of the two proportions (for categorical data). A straight line, going through the value for the standardized difference and the level of power desired, gives the required total sample size for a significance level of 0.01 or 0.05.

Prediction   Forecast of the value for a variable, based on knowledge of the value of at least one other variable, and a **model** which links the former (**outcome variable**) to the latter (**predictor variable**).

Predictive values	In the context of **diagnostic testing**, predictive values measure how useful a test is in practice. The positive predictive value (PPV) of a test is the probability of actually having a condition *given* that the test result is positive. The negative predictive value (NPV) is the probability of not having the disease *given* that the test is negative. From Table 2 (p 36):

$$PPV = \frac{\text{all testing positive and diseased}}{\text{all testing positive}} = \frac{a}{a+b}$$

$$NPV = \frac{\text{all testing negative and non-diseased}}{\text{all testing negative}} = \frac{d}{c+d}$$

Predictive values are affected by changes in the **prevalence** of a condition. A lower prevalence results in a decreased PPV, and a higher prevalence results in an increased PPV. The opposite is true for the NPV. Thus, good diagnostic tools (in terms of **sensitivity** and **specificity**) may lead to a large number of false positive diagnoses in circumstances of low disease prevalence.

Predictor variable	*x*, explanatory or independent variable. In the context of **regression**, it refers to a variable used to determine or **predict** the values of another variable called the **outcome**.

Pretest probability	In the context of **diagnostic testing**, the probability that an individual patient has got a disease or condition *prior* to the undertaking of relevant diagnostic procedures. The pretest probability of having a disease is usually estimated by the **prevalence** of the disease. The following formula is used to convert pretest probabilities (*p*) into pretest odds:

$$\text{Pretest odds} = \frac{p}{1-p} \quad \left(\text{and } p = \frac{\text{odds}}{1+\text{odds}}\right)$$

Likelihood ratios are used to convert pretest odds into posttest odds, which in turn can give the **posttest probability** of disease. See Box 20 (p 60) for an example of these calculations.

Prevalence	Measure of morbidity or disease occurrence. As opposed to **incidence**, it is the total number of *existing* cases of a disease or condition at a particular point in time (point prevalence) or during some specified period (period prevalence), divided by the total population or by the total population at mid-point of the specified interval. Usually expressed as a percentage or per 1000, 10 000 or 100 000 if very small. In the context of **diagnostic testing**, prevalence is often used as an estimate of the **pretest probability** of disease.

Principal components analysis	**Multivariate method** of data reduction in which the original measurements of several variables are replaced by their weighted averages, the 'principal components'. These are termed first, second, etc., and should be uncorrelated with each other. The first principal component is the one which maximizes differences between subjects. The *eigenvalue* is a measure of the amount of variation explained by each principal component. A plot of eigenvalues vs component number is used to decide on the number of principal components to retain. The analysis may provide a single index that uses information contained in all the variables considered.
Prognostic factors	Patient or disease characteristics which influence the course of a particular condition.
Proportion	Ratio of the number of subjects with a given characteristic to the total number of subjects in a group.
Prospective study	**Follow-up** or longitudinal study in which data on **exposure** are first collected, and subjects are followed up for the development of a given condition or **outcome**. **Cohort studies** and **clinical trials** are in this category. The term is also used to refer to a study which uses newly collected data, as opposed to existing information. In this sense, **case-control studies** can sometimes be carried out prospectively, in particular case-control studies which are nested in cohort studies.
Publication bias	Type of **bias** which arises due to selective publication in medical journals of articles which report **statistically significant** results. Given that statistical significance is not synonymous with quality, **validity (2)**, or **clinical significance**, this practice can cause studies of poor quality and misleading results to have much greater impact on clinical and policy decisions than they merit. Also, good studies which have conclusively demonstrated a lack of treatment effect or a lack of association may never get to be published. The importance of such studies is often underestimated. If a study has been planned and conducted in an appropriate way, to provide answers to important questions, the results it produces are both reliable and important, regardless of the magnitude or significance of the same. The issue of publication bias is central to **systematic reviews**, which should not be conducted without an exhaustive search for all published and unpublished studies on the particular subject of interest.

Qualitative variable	See **categorical variable**.
Quantitative variable	Count (**discrete variable**, e.g. number of children, number of times visited doctor, etc.) or measurement (**continuous variable**, e.g. height, body mass index, etc.). For such variables, there is usually a true zero representing the absence of a quantity or a zero count, and in addition, it is sensible to talk about doubling or halving the measurements or counts. See also **interval** and **ratio variables**.
Quartiles	For a given variable sorted in ascending order, the 25th **percentile** or lower quartile is the value below which 25% of all observations fall, and the 75th percentile or upper quartile is the value below which 75% of the observations fall. The range of values falling between the two quartiles is known as the **interquartile range** (Figure 4, p 8).
R-squared (r^2)	The square of the **Pearson's correlation coefficient**. Used in the context of **correlation** and **regression**, it represents the proportion of total **variability** in a variable (the **outcome** in regression) which is explained by another variable or variables (**predictors** in regression). In other words, it states how much of the value of one of the variables can be attributed *solely* to the value of the other variable(s). It is a useful way of assessing the **clinical significance** of the association between two or more variables. A better measure is the adjusted r^2, which is corrected for chance predictions, thus enabling the comparison of regression **models** with different number of predictor variables. For the relationship depicted on Figure 15, p 67, r^2 is equal to 0.17, i.e. 17% of the variability found in bone density can be explained by age.
Random	The quality of something which has no defined pattern. Term commonly used in the context of **sampling** (selecting a study **sample**) to refer to a sample which is not **biased**, and therefore does not display any patterns or trends which are different from those displayed by its source **population**.
Random allocation	See **randomization**.
Random effects	As opposed to **fixed effects**. Term used in the context of **meta-analysis**, when results from individual studies are combined producing a single

estimate. Confidence intervals for these estimates are computed by adding *extra* uncertainty (random effect) to that which is always associated with estimation. The assumption is that the studies being summarized are just a random sample of all possible studies, the underlying 'true' value for the **population** varying from study to study. Tests of **heterogeneity** are used to decide on the choice of a random or fixed effects model. In the context of **analysis of variance**, the term is used to refer to factors (e.g. subject or observer) whose values do not take fixed values (unlike gender, for example), since in studies where subjects and observers are factors, different groups of subjects or observers can be used.

Random-ization
Process of allocating treatment units (patients) to the alternative treatments in a **clinical trial**. The purpose of randomization is to produce comparable treatment groups, with respect to important **prognostic factors**. Randomization is therefore one of the main ways of avoiding **selection biases**. One of its main advantages is that treatment allocation can be carried out **blindly**, before patient entry into a trial, i.e. without knowledge of who the patients may be, the order in which patients will appear or the treatments to which they are being allocated. This can be done by preparing a randomization list using random numbers, either from tables or computer generated. Simple random allocation does not always produce the desired effects, especially when **sample sizes** are small. Modifications to the simple procedure are sometimes necessary. **Minimization** is a *quasi*-random allocation procedure which ensures similar distribution of important prognostic factors in the treatment groups, and is especially good for small samples. Stratified random allocation (within groups of patients with similar characteristics) is used to the same effect, especially with larger samples. Random allocation may sometimes produce groups with unequal sample sizes. This problem may be eliminated by using **restricted randomization**.

Randomized controlled trial (RCT)
Clinical trial where at least two treatment groups are compared, one of them serving as the **control** group, and treatment allocation is carried out using a **random, unbiased** method.

Range
Interval that goes from the minimum to the maximum value in a set of **quantitative** measurements. Commonly reported as a single figure, e.g. 6, preferably, both the minimum and maximum should be quoted (e.g. 11 to 17).

Rank correlation	**Non-parametric method** of assessing the association between **quantitative** or between **ordinal variables. Spearman's** and **Kendall's rank correlation** are the methods commonly employed. The resulting coefficients (ρ and τ) are to be interpreted in the same way as the **Pearson's correlation coefficient**. However, rank correlation methods assess linear relationships between the **ranks** given to the values of the variables in question (see Figure 18, p 77).

Ranks
The relative position of the observations in a given variable (**ordinal** or **interval/ratio**). For example, if one had the variable 'age', in years, with five observations: 65, 49, 31, 57 and 49 (reordered: 31, 49, 49, 57, 65), these would be given the ranks: 1, 2.5, 2.5, 4 and 5. When values are ordered according to size into a 'league table', the rank of a given value represents its position in the table. **Non-parametric methods** of analysis are frequently based on ranks.

Rate
Summary measure which conveys the idea of **risk** over time. The denominator is expressed as **person-time at risk** and the numerator is the number of new occurrences of a particular event. Rates can be used as measures of mortality (mortality rates) or morbidity (**incidence rates**).

Rate ratio
Ratio of the **rate** of an event in one group (**exposure** or intervention) to that in another group (**control**). It is one of the **relative risk** measures commonly used in research studies. If there is no difference between the rates in the two groups, the rate ratio will be 1. A rate ratio greater than 1 suggests a greater event rate in the exposure group. The opposite is true if the rate ratio is less than 1. From Table 1 (p 15):

$$\text{Rate ratio} = \frac{a/\text{PTAR in the exposed}}{b/\text{PTAR in the unexposed}}$$

where PTAR is the **person-time at risk** in each group.

Ratio variable
Quantitative variable which has a true zero. Unlike **interval variables**, the ratio of two values has the same meaning regardless of the scale used to make the measurements. An example of this type of variable is weight. A 10% increase in weight from 30 to 33 pounds still corresponds to the same 10% increase when measurements are expressed in kilograms (approximately from 13.6 to 15.0 kg).

RCT
See **randomized controlled trial**.

Recall bias   See **information bias**.

Reference   Range of values which measures the **variability** of a given measurement
range   among 'normal' individuals (thus, sometimes called 'normal range').
'Normal' usually refers to non-diseased individuals, but the definition of
'normal' may vary with the context in which it is used. Thus, a clear
description of the characteristics of the **sample** used to construct any
reference range is very important. Within a 95% reference range we find
95% of all individual observations for a given measurement, 2.5% lying
outside of either limit of the range. To be sure this range is calculated with a
fair degree of certainty, it is important to have a large enough **sample size**
(some authors suggest at least 200). If the measurements follow an
approximate **normal distribution**, their **mean** and **standard deviation** can
be used to construct the reference range:

95% Reference range = mean $\pm 1.96 \times$ SD

Reference ranges can also be constructed using the relevant **percentiles** of
the distribution of the variable in question (e.g. the 2.5th and the 97.5th
percentiles for a 95% reference range). This does not require that the data
are normally distributed.

Regression   Statistical method used especially for the purpose of **prediction**. In simple
linear regression, the relationship between the **outcome variable (y)** and the
predictor variable (x), both **interval/ratio**, is summarized by means of a
model or line. Figure 15 shows the regression of bone density (in arbitrary
study units) on age (in years) in postmenopausal women, from the example
in Box 2 (see model in Box 12, p 43), as a weak to moderate negative

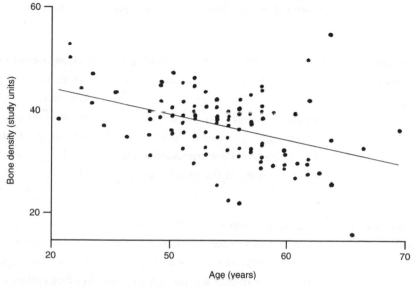

Figure 15   Graphical display of a regression analysis.

association. The regression model is used to predict the value of the outcome variable given the value of the predictor. In other words, the model specifies by how much the value of y will go up (or down) for each unit increase in the value of x. 'By how much' is given by the **regression coefficient** or slope of the best fit line. Another characteristic of this line is the **intercept**, i.e. the predicted value for y when x is equal to zero. The line of best fit is found using the **least squares** method, which seeks to minimize the total sum of the squared differences (i.e. *vertical* distances or **residuals**) from each observation to any given straight line going through the data points. Residuals are used to assess the **goodness-of-fit** of regression models. **Categorical** predictors may also be included in regression models, either on their own (equivalent to **analysis of variance**) or together with **quantitative** predictors (**analysis of covariance**). Generally, **multiple regression** allows the use of more than one predictor variable. When the outcomes are categorical, **logistic regression** is indicated. **Cox regression** is used for the analysis of **survival** times and **Poisson regression** to analyse counts and **rates**.

Regression coefficient	or slope of the line of best fit. It represents the increments predicted in the **outcome variable** for each unit increase in the **predictor variable** (Box 12, p 43). When the predictor is a **categorical variable** the regression coefficient represents the average difference between any given level of the variable and the level taken as the baseline or standard (e.g. smokers vs non-smokers; see Box 2, p 3). As with the **correlation coefficient (r)**, a slope of 0 represents no relationship between the variables. However, regression coefficients are not restricted to take values between -1 and $+1$. In theory, they can take any value from $-\infty$ to $+\infty$: unlike r, which is 'unitless', regression coefficients are expressed in the same units as the outcome variable.
Regression diagnostics	Checks carried out after developing a **regression model** in order to assess the suitability of the same model. One important aspect concerns the **assumption** of a linear relationship between **outcome** and **predictor variable**. The presence of **outlying** or extreme observations may exert undue influence on a regression model. Plots of **residuals** are widely used to detect these situations. Data **transformations** (e.g. to a logarithmic scale) can often deal with many of the problems encountered.
Relative risk (RR)	**Summary measure** which represents the ratio of the risk of a given event in one group of subjects compared to another group, where risk broadly represents **risk, rate** or **odds**. It is sometimes used as a synonym for **risk ratio**, but in its broad sense it also refers to **odds ratios** and **rate ratios**. When the 'risk' of the event of interest is the same in the two groups, the

relative risk is 1. It will be less than 1 if the group represented in the numerator is at a lower 'risk' of the event, and greater than 1 if the opposite is true.

Relative risk reduction (RRR)

Alternative way of expressing **relative risk (RR)**. It is calculated as follows:

$$RRR = (1 - RR) \times 100\%$$

The RRR can be interpreted as the **proportion** of the initial or baseline 'risk' which was eliminated by a given treatment or intervention, or by avoidance of **exposure** to a **risk factor** (Box 22). When the RR gives values greater than 1, what is calculated is the 'excess relative risk':

$$ERR = (RR - 1) \times 100\%$$

BOX 22
From **Box 1**, p 1. The RR for the effect of aspirin relative to no aspirin is 0.80 and the RRR is 20%. **Interpretation:** The risk of vascular death in the aspirin group, at 5 weeks, is 80% of the risk in the control group, and therefore, aspirin reduced the risk of vascular death at 5 weeks by 20%.

Reliability

In the context of clinical measurement. Quality of a method of measurement which consistently gives the same results. Thus, reliability requires **repeatability** (when measurement is repeated under the same conditions), and **reproducibility** (when measurement is repeated under different conditions). An index of reliability (R) can be calculated from the **variability** of the repeated (or paired) measurements (see repeatability):

$$R = 1 - \frac{\text{observed disagreement}}{\text{chance-expected disagreement}}$$

where observed disagreement = 'variance of errors' (see repeatability) and chance-expected disagreement = **variance** of all measurements, ignoring the pairing (DUNN and EVERITT, 1995). R takes values from 0 (no reliability) to 1 (perfect reliability). There is a parallel between this measure of 'agreement' for **quantitative** measurements and the **kappa statistic** used to assess agreement between measurements on a **categorical** scale: R measures the proportion of the observed variability in the measurements which is over and above that due to measurement error (i.e. the proportion which is due to variability in the subjects being studied). R (like *kappa*) is population-dependent. For the same measuring device or method, the value of R will vary according to the variance of the measurements in different populations.

Greater variability has the effect of increasing the value of R (reliability can be thought of as repeatability put into context: if a measurement has little variability in a population, there is less acceptance of poor repeatability, but if it varies considerably, one is less stringent). The reliability of a measuring method gives information on how good the method is at ascribing the correct measurement value to individuals in a population. Another measure of reliability is the **intraclass correlation coefficient**. See Appendix D for a worked example.

Repeatability

In the context of clinical measurement, it refers to the **variability** of **repeated measurements** taken under *similar* conditions. Repeatability can be expressed by the **standard deviation (SD)** of the measurement errors (sometimes called 'standard error of measurement'):

$$SD \text{ of errors} = \sqrt{\text{variance of errors}}$$

$$\text{Variance of errors} = \frac{\sum(\text{differences})^2}{2n}$$

where $\sum$ represents summation, and difference = measurement$_1$ − measurement$_2$ (DUNN and EVERITT, 1995). The SD of errors can be used to calculate, say, 95% 'limits of agreement' for the repeatability of a given measurement. Their interpretation is similar to that of **reference ranges**. The **estimate** of the SD of errors should therefore come from a large **unbiased sample** of individuals. Repeatability is important in the assessment of **reliability** (in the formula for R, observed disagreement = variance of errors). See Appendix D for a worked example.

Repeated measurements analysis

Analysis of measurements taken on one or more groups of subjects, where more than one measurement per subject is taken, usually over a period of time. The main issue here is the lack of **independence** of observations pertaining to a single subject. Data of this sort are commonly analysed using inadequate methods (including incorrect graphical displays), such as **multiple significance testing** (multiple comparisons at different time points), **analysis of variance** in which the lack of independence of the observations is not taken into account, and graphs showing the average for each group at the different time points, thus 'hiding' possibly important individual patterns. Although special repeated measures analysis of variance methods do exist, which deal with the above problems, other straightforward and effective methods may also be used, requiring solely the choice of sensible **summary measures**. These summaries reduce the multiplicity of data to fewer 'observations' (the chosen summaries), which in turn may be analysed by simple methods. For example, heart rate measurements over a period of 3 h (measured at 10-min intervals – 18 measurements per patient), following the administration of two different anxiolytic drugs, may be averaged, producing a single posttreatment measurement for each patient in the trial. An example of a correct graphical display can be found in Figure 2 (p 5), where the pattern of response over time is presented for each subject separately.

Reproducibility

In the context of clinical measurement, it refers to the **variability** of repeated measurements taken under *different* conditions, for example, the comparison of two alternative methods of measurement. **Repeatability** within *each* method is an important determinant of reproducibility, and should always be assessed. See ALTMAN (1991) or BLAND and ALTMAN (1986) for worked examples.

Residuals

In the context of **regression**, residuals are the numerical differences between observed and **predicted** values. The analysis of the pattern of residuals is useful in determining the appropriateness of a particular **model** to the data it proposes to describe (**regression diagnostics**).

Restricted randomization

Treatment allocation method which aims to produce treatment groups with equal number of subjects. CAMPBELL and MACHIN (1993) give an example of a trial where two treatments, A and B, are compared. Blocks of four patients are generated, to include all possible combinations of the two treatments that give equal allocation. In this case six possible combinations are generated:

1	AABB	4	BABA
2	ABAB	5	BAAB
3	ABBA	6	BBAA

A sequence of **random** digits is generated (e.g. 225, 673, 451), to represent the combinations that will be used. The above sequence gives the following treatment allocation for the first 12 patients:

ABABABABBAAB ...

The end result is treatment groups with equal **sample sizes**.

Retrospective study

Observational study in which information on **outcome** (presence or absence of disease) is first collected, and subjects are subsequently investigated (usually by interview or by looking at employment or other records) for possible past **exposure** to a **risk factor** of interest. **Case-control studies** are in this category. The term is also used to refer to a study which uses data collected prior to the set up of the investigation, as opposed to newly collected data. In this sense, **cohort studies** can sometimes be carried out retrospectively.

Risk

Probability of occurrence of a given event. Calculated as:

$$\text{Risk} = \frac{\text{number of events}}{\text{number of people at risk}}$$

Risk factors

Factors, in particular patient characteristics, history of disease, family history, occupational exposure, and socioeconomic and demographic factors, which increase an individual's probability of disease when compared to individuals in whom the factors in question are absent. See also **exposure**.

Risk ratio

Ratio of the **risk** of an event in one group (**exposure** or intervention) to that in another group (**control**). The term **relative risk** is sometimes used as a synonym of risk ratio. If there is no difference in risk between the two groups, the risk ratio will be 1. A risk ratio greater than 1 suggests a greater risk of the event in the exposure group. The opposite is true if the risk ratio is less than 1. From Table 1 (p 15):

$$\text{Risk ratio} = \frac{\text{risk in exposed group}}{\text{risk in control group}} = \frac{a}{(a+c)} \div \frac{b}{(b+d)}$$

Robust method

Descriptive term for a measure, **significance test** or method of **estimation** which is not grossly affected by influential **outlying** observations. **Medians**, **confidence intervals** based on **ranks** and **non-parametric tests** are common examples.

ROC curve

or receiver operating characteristic curve. Graphical display of the performance of a **quantitative diagnostic test**. The graph is a plot of **sensitivity** or detection rate vs false positive rate (100−**specificity**%), for selected cut-off points. This enables the comparison of the performance of different cut points to be made. The choice of cut point above which disease is considered to be present is made taking into account the trade-off between false positive and false negative rates. A good cut-off point should be close to the top left hand corner of the graph: high detection rate, low false positive rate. The graph in Figure 16 shows the performance of hCG (human chorionic gonadotrophin) in **screening** for Down's syndrome. Quantitative

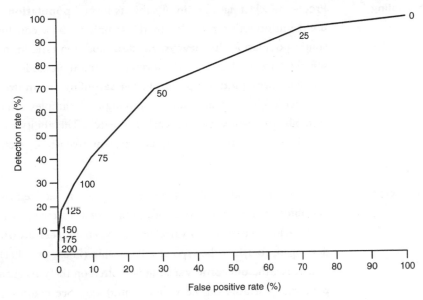

Figure 16 ROC curve for hCG: screening for Down's syndrome (Oxford–Barts data set used with kind permission of Professor Nicholas Wald, Wolfson Institute of Preventive Medicine, London).

measurements need not always be dichotomized into disease present/absent, since the calculation of **likelihood ratios** permits a better use of the spectrum of values obtained by the diagnostic test.

Sample   Group of subjects selected or **sampled** from a wider group or **population** according to some prespecified criteria. Samples are used in research studies to **estimate** population parameters, and thus, it is important for samples to be representative of their source population, and of adequate **size.**

Sample size (required)   Number of subjects required in a study so that differences thought to be **clinically important** can also be detected as **statistically significant** (at a given level of α or **type I error**), if indeed they do exist. In some instances, sample sizes are calculated for the purpose of **estimation**, in which case the issue is not **power** but the **precision (2)** (or width) of **confidence intervals** constructed around the observed quantities (**means, proportions,** differences, etc.). Such calculations produce larger required sample sizes, as compared to 'power calculations'. A few formulae and a worked example for sample size calculations are presented in Appendix B. KIRKWOOD (1988) gives formulae for a number of **summary measures** for both power and precision calculations. CLINSTAT (BLAND, 1991) performs a number of power calculations.

Sampling	Process of selecting a group of subjects from a **population**, with the aim to use the information provided by the sample to draw conclusions about the source population. In **surveys**, **random** and non-random methods of sampling are used. Among the former, common methods are simple random sampling, **stratified sampling**, **cluster sampling** and **multistage sampling**. Systematic sampling and quota sampling are examples of non-random methods, frequently used in market research. The ability to generalize from sample to population relies on its representativeness or lack of **bias**.
Scatterplot	Graphical method for displaying the association between two **quantitative variables**. It is always a good idea to present a scatterplot when assessing the **correlation** between two variables, or when **regression models** are developed, to assess the type of relationship (linear or other) present. In the latter case, the **outcome variable** is plotted on the y-(vertical) axis, and the **predictor variable** on the x-(horizontal) axis. See Figures 14 and 15 on pp 56 and 67.
Screening	Clinical, laboratory, radiological or other tests, carried out for the purpose of identifying risk factors for disease. This is usually done on 'healthy' individuals. For example, pregnant women may be screened for high hCG levels as a **risk factor** for carrying a Down's syndrome fetus. If levels are found to be high, it is still necessary to run **diagnostic tests** to establish the presence of Down's syndrome (amniocentesis for chromosome typing).
SD	See **standard deviation**.
SE	See **standard error**.
Selection bias	In the context of **surveys**, selection **bias** refers to systematic differences between a **sample** and its source **population**, usually caused by inappropriate **sampling** (sampling bias). Conclusions drawn from such a sample are unlikely to be generalizable to the entire population. **Case-control studies** are also prone to selection bias: cases who have higher levels of **exposure** are more likely to be diagnosed in the first place, and therefore to be included in studies. This happens because their unusually high levels of exposure to a particular **risk factor** result in more intensive investigation (detection bias) when they present their complaints to a doctor. In the context of **clinical trials**, selection biases occur due to methods of treatment allocation which lead to imbalances between treatment groups, with respect

to important **prognostic factors** (allocation bias). Problems occurring after patient entry into a trial may also lead to selection biases (**drop-outs**, **'cross-overs'**, **withdrawals**, etc.).

Sensitivity

or detection rate. In the context of **diagnostic testing**, it measures how good a test is in detecting those individuals who are truly diseased or have some condition (true positives). From Table 2 (p 36):

$$\text{Sensitivity} = \frac{\text{all testing positive and diseased}}{\text{all diseased}} = \frac{a}{a+c}$$

The complement of sensitivity is the false negative rate: $c/(a+c)$. Like **specificity**, sensitivity is usually not affected by changes in **prevalence** of the condition in question. However, it can be affected by **spectrum bias**. Use of the term detection rate is more intuitive and should be encouraged.

Sensitivity analysis

Repetition of a particular statistical procedure or calculation, under different assumptions, to assess the impact of each of these assumptions or scenarios on the results of a study, or on the logistic requirements for an investigation. For example, in a **follow-up study**, statistical analysis is first carried out with the data available, which excludes data from patients lost to follow-up, and then repeated to include all subjects originally in the study. **Outcomes** for the missing observations are imputed, allowing for the best or worst scenarios, as appropriate to the aims of the study in question. This second analysis of the data may yield results which are not consistent with the previous analysis. In such cases, the results first obtained should be carefully considered. In terms of study requirements, sensitivity analysis can be used, for example, to calculate the **sample sizes required** given different scenarios, where either of the following may change: **type I error**, **power** of the study, ratio between number of unexposed and **exposed**, expected differences between groups, degree of **variability** of measurements, etc. In **meta-analysis**, in which some individual studies may be of poorer quality than others, sensitivity analysis is used to assess the impact of removing such studies from the analysis.

Shapiro–Wilk test

Significance test used to assess departures from a **normal distribution** for **quantitative variables**. If the Shapiro–Wilk test for a given variable gives a small **P-value** (say, <0.05), the assumption of normality is usually rejected. A statistic frequently reported in addition to the test statistic W is V, which takes the value of 1 if a variable has a normal distribution, or greater than 1 if not. An equivalent test is the Shapiro–Francia test.

Significance tests	Tests which are performed with the purpose of assessing the plausibility of a given study hypothesis. These hypotheses stem from questions such as 'are smokers at greater risk of having lung cancer?', 'is drug A better than drug B in treating asthma?', etc. The test assesses the compatibility of the data collected in the study with the **null hypothesis**. A **P-value** is produced, which gives the probability of the observed result, or a more extreme result, under the null hypothesis. A problem-oriented summary of statistical tests commonly used is presented in Appendix B.
Simple regression	**Regression** in which a single **predictor variable** is used in a **model** predicting an **outcome**.
Skewness	The quality of a **distribution** which has a relatively long left (negatively skewed) or right (positively skewed) hand tail (Figure 17). Positively skewed distributions can sometimes be converted into **normal distributions** by taking logs of the original values. Such variables are said to have a **lognormal distribution**. Alternatively, data which display a skew can be analysed using **non-parametric methods**, which make no **assumptions** about the distribution of the variable(s) in question.

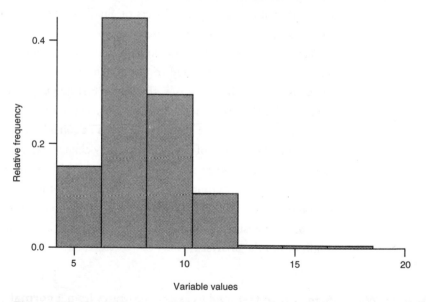

Figure 17 Positively skewed distribution.

Slope	See **regression coefficient**.
SMR	See **standardized mortality ratio**.

Spearman's
rho
(ρ)

Non-parametric correlation coefficient which is calculated by computing the **Pearson's correlation coefficient** for the association between the **ranks** given to the values of the variables involved, as opposed to the actual data values. It can be used with **interval/ratio** data which do not meet the requirements for Pearson's correlation, or with **ordinal** data. Figure 18 shows the same graph presented in Figure 14 (p 56), but a few fictitious **outliers** were included. In this situation, the non-parametric correlation coefficient gives a better estimate of the true relationship between bone density and age.

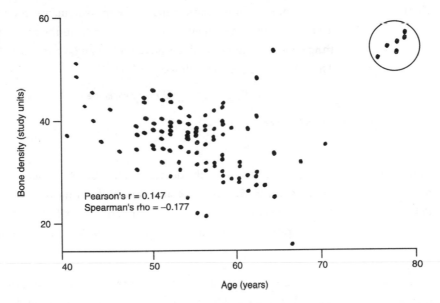

Figure 18   Spearman's rank correlation on data with outliers.

Specificity

In the context of **diagnostic testing**, it measures how good a test is in detecting those individuals who are not diseased or do not have some condition (true negatives). From Table 2 (p 36):

$$\text{Specificity} = \frac{\text{all testing negative and non-diseased}}{\text{all non-diseased}} = \frac{b}{b+d}$$

The complement of specificity is the false positive rate (FPR): $b/(b+d)$. Like **sensitivity**, specificity is not usually affected by changes in **prevalence**. However, it can be affected by **spectrum bias**. The concept of false positive rate is more intuitive than that of specificity. In addition, the false positive rate readily gives useful information: one may not have the feel for the difference between a test that has 98% specificity and one that has 96%. However, when expressed as FPRs (2% vs 4%), it is clear that one of the tests produces *twice* the number of false positives.

Spectrum bias	**Bias** which occurs when estimating the **sensitivity** and **specificity** of a **diagnostic test**, in groups of patients with different severity of disease. Spectrum bias may explain why different studies, evaluating the same diagnostic test, give different results. This type of bias is sometimes overlooked given the widespread belief that the sensitivity and specificity of a diagnostic test are immutable properties of the test.
Standard deviation (SD)	Measure of the spread or **variability** of a set of measurements. Usually employed in conjunction with the **mean** to describe **interval/ratio** data. The SD is expressed in the same units as the measurements in question. It is the average distance individual observations are from the mean. **Reference ranges**, which are useful descriptive tools, can be constructed using the SD. The SD is calculated as follows: $$SD = \sqrt{variance}$$ (see **variance**).
Standard error (SE)	Statistic which indicates the degree of uncertainty in calculating an **estimate** from a **sample**. **Sample size** and **variability** of measurements are the main determinants of the magnitude of standard errors. Standard errors are more easily interpreted when used to construct **confidence intervals**.
Standard-ization	Statistical method used to compare **rates** in different **populations**. The rationale for standardization is the potential for **confounding**, which exists in many **observational studies**, and may lead to **biased** or erroneous results. Standardization is usually performed to adjust for differences in age and sex distribution in the populations being compared. Direct and indirect standardization methods are used (BLAND, 1995). The former is used when studying large populations, and it involves the calculation of **standardized event rates** (commonly age-standardized). These are calculated by applying the **age-specific rates** observed in the study population (for example, the population in a particular country, region or town) to the age structure (i.e. proportion in each age group) of some prespecified standard population (for example, the population in England and Wales is often used as the standard population in studies looking at different regional health authorities). In the indirect method, the number of **expected** events in the study population is calculated, under the assumption that each age group in this population has experienced the same mortality or morbidity rates as the standard population. The ratio between observed and expected number of events produces a standardized event ratio (e.g. **standardized mortality ratio** or **SMR**). The study population can now be compared either to the standard

population, or to another study population whose SMR has been computed using the same standard population. This method is especially appropriate for the study of small study populations, since the study population's event rates for the different age groups will not be **estimated** with enough **precision (2)**. It these cases it is preferable to work with the event rates for the standard population.

Standardized event rate

Adjusted mortality or morbidity **rate** (commonly age and sex adjusted) obtained using direct **standardization** methods. The adjusted event rate is calculated by adding all age or age/sex-specific adjusted rates, computed by applying the standard age/sex specific rates to the study population's age/sex structure, to produce a single overall measure of what the event rate would be in the study population, if it had the same age/sex structure as the standard population.

Standardized mortality ratio (SMR)

Ratio between observed and **expected** numbers of an event (death or other), multiplied by 100:

$$SMR = \frac{observed}{expected} \times 100$$

SMRs are computed by indirect **standardization**. An SMR of 100 suggests the **rate** of occurrence of the event in the study population is the same as in the standard/base population.

Statistical significance

Refers to the result of a **significance test**, when the associated **P-value** is found to be below a predetermined (but arbitrary) cut-off point, conventionally set at $P = 0.05$. For correct interpretation, it is good practice to avoid expressions such as '$P < 0.05$' or 'NS (non-significant)' when reporting the results of a test, and to quote exact P-values instead. In addition, **confidence intervals** should always be obtained for an assessment of the **clinical significance** of the study results.

Statistical tests

See **significance tests**.

Stepwise regression

Method of selection of variables to be included as **predictors** in **multiple regression models**. This can be carried out as forward or backward selection, and most statistical packages will perform the procedure in an automated way. The rationale behind it is the need to find predictors which relate independently to the **outcome variable**, and to simplify explanatory or predictive models, thus avoiding complex, unstable models, with highly correlated and redundant predictor variables. When conducting an investigation, researchers collect information on several potential explanatory variables, and may start data analysis by finding which of these is most strongly associated with the response variable (forward selection). The **residuals** resulting from fitting a model with just this one variable are then correlated with the other predictor variables in turn, the one most strongly correlated with the residuals being added to the model. These steps are repeated until no more variables are found to make a **statistically significant** contribution to the model. In backward elimination, all variables are included and subsequently dropped from the model if found to make no contribution to it. Best sub-sets regression is possibly a better alternative to stepwise methods, but fewer statistical packages perform this method. Because models are developed on the basis of data observed in a particular **sample,** they need to be validated against an **independent** set of data, or against a **random** sub-set of the study data (not used to develop the model).

Strata

Levels of a **categorical variable** (or categorized **quantitative variable**). Each *stratum* corresponds to a single level or to a combination of levels of two or more factors. An example of *strata* are age and age/sex groups.

Stratification

Computation of **estimates** or **significance tests** for each *stratum* of a classifying variable. The rationale for stratification is **confounding.** Results from each *stratum* are summarized to produce single estimates or single test statistics across all *strata*. The **Mantel–Haenszel chi-squared test** and **Mantel–Haenszel estimates** are methods commonly used to obtain overall tests of significance, and to pool estimates across *strata*. See Box 4, (p 14), for an example.

Stratified sampling

Method of **sampling** which aims to produce a **sample** that is representative of all *strata* in a given **population.** This is usually done by choosing the same proportion of individuals from each *stratum* so that the structure in the population is replicated in the sample.

Study design

Chosen method of collecting the information necessary to answer a particular research question. It involves decisions on whether to intervene actively (**clinical trial**) or simply describe what is observed (**observational study**), on the timing for collecting information on **exposure** and **outcome** (**follow-up** or **case-control study**), on the choice of **controls** (**parallel** or **crossover design**), the required **sample size**, etc.

Subgroup analyses

Testing of study hypotheses in subgroups of patients with common characteristics (e.g. females, elderly, patients with onset of acute myocardial infarction <12 h, etc.), with the view to assess the magnitude and significance of treatment effects in those same subgroups, or to make comparisons with other subgroups. Although there is a justifiable clinical interest in doing so, such analyses are seldom carried out in an appropriate way. In particular, the issues of adequate **sample size** and **multiple significance testing** should be considered at the planning stages. Also, the comparison of subgroups based on the comparison of **P-values** (obtained from within-group analyses) should be discouraged in favour of correctly testing for **interaction** (i.e. interaction between the 'treatment' and the characteristic defining the 'subgroups', for example, age group).

Summary measures

or summary statistics, such as **means, proportions, standard deviation, regression coefficients, relative risks**, etc., which reduce the information contained in several data values into a single value. Summary measures are frequently used in the analysis of **repeated measurements**. In this context, the choice of summary will depend on the way the variable of interest changes with time. MATTHEWS *et al.* (1990) divide this broadly into 'peaked' and 'growth' patterns, and give summaries which are appropriate in each circumstance. The **area under the curve** is one such measure, normally used when the mean is inappropriate.

Surveillance bias

See **information bias**.

Surveys

Observational studies aimed at describing one or more characteristics of a given population. These can be the **prevalence** of a disease or the average value of a given measurement. Surveys are usually conducted by studying a **cross-section** of the **target population**. **Random sampling** is of paramount importance in the conduct of surveys, to ensure **sample** representativeness.

Survival analysis

Analysis of survival studies (where the **outcome** may be death or any other event of interest), usually concerned with **predicting** length of survival given a number of characteristics or **prognostic factors**, or with comparing the survival experiences of two or more groups of individuals. **Censoring** occurs frequently in this type of study, whereby the outcome for some individuals is not known at the end of the study period. Duration of **follow-up** may also be different from subject to subject. Thus, methods used for **proportions** (e.g. 'what proportion of people died after 3 years?') or methods for **quantitative data** (e.g. 'what was the mean length of survival?') should not be used. The

log rank test is used for making comparisons between groups. In addition, **Cox regression** produces predictive **models**. Other methods of analysis include the construction of **life tables** and survival curves (**Kaplan–Meier method**). When planning a survival study, it must be considered that the **sample size required** depends on the number of events, and the rate at which they are expected to occur in the accrual and follow-up periods.

Systematic review

Review of the methods and results from all individual studies which focus on a particular research question and conform to set criteria. The term encompasses the whole process of doing a systematic review, i.e. identification and selection of studies, assessment of their validity, and description of results. It also includes the use of special statistical methods to obtain overall single **estimates** (for example, of the effect of a particular treatment versus a placebo) known as **meta-analysis. Publication bias** may be a problem when conducting systematic reviews or overviews. CHALMERS and ALTMAN (eds, 1995) give a broad discussion of issues around systematic reviews.

t-tests

Significance tests used to compare the **means** of two different groups. **Paired** or **independent** samples t-tests are appropriate depending on **study design**. The number of **degrees of freedom** for the independent samples test is $N - 2$, where N is the total sample size, $n_1 + n_2$. Both the test statistic and the corresponding degrees of freedom are referred to tables of the t-distribution for assessment of **statistical significance**. An **assumption** of the independent samples t-test is that the variable of interest has a **normal distribution** and similar **variance** in the two groups being compared. Modifications to the standard test allow for unequal variances. See Appendix C for a worked example.

Target population

Population to whom the results of a given investigation (based on a **sample** of subjects drawn from the population in question) are to be generalized. A distinction is usually made between the wider target population, and the study population, this being a subset of the former, used to select the study sample.

Transform-ations

Data manipulations which attempt to find the right measurement scale, usually for variables which are not **normally distributed. Parametric methods** of analysis can then be used on the transformed data. In particular, data with a positive **skew** may benefit from a logarithmic transformation. **Geometric means** (Figure 7, p 27) are then calculated by backtransforming the arithmetic mean of the values on the log scale. Another common transformation is the logit, in the context of **logistic regression**.

Treatment-period interaction	In the context of **crossover trials**, this type of interaction occurs when the differences observed between any two treatments vary, depending on whether the comparison is made in the first or in the second period of the trial (in the case of a two-period trial). This is usually due to the effect of the treatment given in the first period being **carried-over** into the second period. Thus, in planning crossover trials, it is important to allow for sufficiently long **wash-out periods** between treatments.
Trend (test for)	Special form of standard **significance tests**, used when the grouping variable is **ordinal**. For example, when assessing the relationship between two **categorical variables**, the **chi-squared test** is normally used. If, however, one of the variables is a **binary variable** and the other is on an ordinal scale ($r \times 2$ **contingency table**), it is of interest to compare not just the **proportions,** but also to look for a trend, i.e. whether the proportions with a particular outcome increase or decrease linearly, across levels of the ordered variable. This is called the chi-squared test for trend, which has one **degree of freedom**. An example would be a cross-tabulation where chronic respiratory disease (yes/no) is the **outcome** and smoking (non-smoker, light smoker, moderate smoker, heavy smoker) represents **exposure**. The questions asked are (a) is the risk of chronic respiratory disease *different* for different types of smokers, and (b) does the risk of chronic respiratory disease *increase* from non-smokers to heavy smokers. The chi-squared trend statistic is always smaller than the standard chi-squared statistic. The difference between the two statistics, on $r - 2$ degrees of freedom, tests the departure from the linear trend (i.e. differences which are not explained by the linear trend). For **quantitative** data, the Cuszick's test, **analysis of variance** (with linear contrasts) or **regression,** can all be used. Non-linear trend (U-shaped curves, for example) can be assessed using regression methods.
Two-by-two (2×2) table	**Contingency table** with two rows and two columns (i.e. four cells).
Two-sided test	**Significance test** which explores both alternative hypotheses to the **null hypothesis**. For example, if making a comparison between the **means** of two groups (e.g. mean cholesterol levels between vegetarians and meat-eaters), the null hypothesis states the two means are the same. The alternative hypothesis, as opposed to that in a **one-sided test**, is that the mean in one of the groups can be either greater *or* smaller than the mean in the other group.

Two-way ANOVA	**Analysis of variance** of data classified according to two factors or characteristics (e.g. ethnic group and gender). Here, the total sum of squares is partitioned between main effects (the factors), and **residual**. When measurements (e.g. blood pressure) are replicated for each subject, it is also possible to check whether there is an **interaction** between the two factors.
Type I error	or α. Probability of failing to accept the **null hypothesis (NH)** when NH is true. See also **P-value**.
Type II error	or β. Probability of failing to reject the **null hypothesis** when the latter is false. This probability becomes smaller with increasing **sample size**. The greater the probability of a type II error, the weaker the **power** of a study to detect differences as **statistically significant** when such differences exist.
Validity (1)	In the context of clinical measurement, this term refers to whether a particular measurement does in fact measure the characteristic which is of interest (for example, does forced expiratory volume at 1 min reflect lung function?). A valid measurement must be **accurate** and **reliable** in order to be useful. However, these are necessary but not sufficient conditions for validity: forced expiratory volume at 1 min could be measured without error and still not reflect lung function.
Validity (2)	This term is also used to refer to a measurement or assessment which is not **biased**. In **surveys**, validity is achieved mainly by **random sampling**, and in **clinical trials** by **randomization**. Randomization ensures the *internal* validity of the results, whereas the composition of the study sample determines the generalizability or *external* validity of the results.
Variability	Variability is present when differences are observed among different individuals or within the same subject, with respect to any characteristic or feature which can be assessed or measured. The main purpose of statistics is to unravel underlying patterns which may be obscured by natural and **random** variation. Commonly used measures of variability or spread are: **standard deviation**, **variance**, **reference range**, **interquartile range**, among others.
Variance	Measure of spread or **variability** of **quantitative** measurements. It is calculated as the sum of the squared differences between individual measurements and the **mean**, divided by the total sample size $(n) - 1$:

$$s^2 = \frac{\text{sum of all squared differences from the mean}}{\text{sample size} - 1} = \frac{\sum(x_i - \bar{x})^2}{n - 1}$$

where x_i is each individual observation and $\bar{x}$ is the mean of all observations. The square root of the variance is the **standard deviation**. [Note: σ^2 is used to refer to the **population** parameter and s^2 to refer to the sample statistic. The latter is used to estimate the former.]

Volunteer bias

Type of bias which occurs particularly in **cross-sectional studies**, when potential participants are asked to provide the information being collected. For example, in a study where questionnaires are sent to all residents of a particular area, or to all patients registered with a given general practice, some individuals will return the study questionnaires (respondents or volunteers) and some people will not (non-respondents). Studies have shown volunteers to be different from non-respondents, in terms of demographic characteristics and **risk factors** for disease (and therefore, likely **outcomes**). Thus, it is important to ensure that non-response is kept at very low levels in this type of investigation.

Wash-out period

In the context of **crossover trials**, it refers to the period of time allowed between two consecutive treatments, to prevent the effect of treatments given in one period being **carried over** into the next period. The effect of the treatments given in the second period can then be assessed independently, without contamination, thus avoiding **treatment-period interactions**.

Wilcoxon matched pairs signed rank test

Non-parametric significance test used to compare **paired ordinal** or **interval/ratio variables** when the **assumptions** for the **paired t-test** cannot be met.

Wilcoxon rank sum test

Significance test which has the same purpose and is mathematically equivalent to the **Mann–Whitney U-test**.

Withdrawals

In the context of **clinical trials,** withdrawals are subjects who do not follow the trial protocol, either because they are withdrawn from the trial by the doctors or researchers conducting the investigation or because the patients themselves choose to drop-out (possibly due to factors associated with the intervention, the disease or the patient). '**Crossovers**' are another example of protocol violation. **Intention-to-treat analysis** minimizes the potential **bias** which arises from these situations.

x-variable	also termed independent, explanatory or **predictor variable**. In **scatterplots** it is plotted on the horizontal axis (ordinate).
y-variable	also termed dependent, response or **outcome variable**. In **scatterplots** it is plotted on the vertical axis (abscissa).
z-scores	Measurements which are expressed in units of **standard deviation (SD)**. For example, if the **mean** height of a group of people is 172 cm with SD equal to 10 cm, a person measuring 182 cm has a z-score of 1 (i.e. +1 SD away from the mean). z-scores are obtained by subtracting the mean from individual measurements (which follow a **normal distribution**), and dividing the result by the SD. The measurements are converted into a distribution with mean 0 and SD 1:

$$z \text{ score} = \frac{\text{observation} - \text{mean}}{\text{SD}}$$

z-test	**Significance test** which is used for comparing **means** or **proportions** between two groups.

Appendix A
Calculating the required sample size: formulae

● **Notation**

n total sample size or sample size for each group if independent samples

σ standard deviation of measurements

σ_w standard deviation of the differences if paired data

δ smallest clinically important difference to be detected

α type I error

β type II error

π proportion

● **Paired samples – difference in means**

$$n = \frac{(z_\alpha + z_{2\beta})^2 \sigma_w^2}{\delta^2}$$

● **Independent samples – difference in means**

$$n = \frac{2(z_\alpha + z_{2\beta})^2 \sigma^2}{\delta^2} \quad \text{per group}$$

● **Independent samples – difference in proportions**

$$n = (z_\alpha + z_{2\beta})^2 [\pi_1(1 - \pi_1) + \pi_2(1 - \pi_2)]/\delta^2 \quad \text{per group}$$

Value for $(z_\alpha + z_{2\beta})^2$ for different values of β ($1 -$ power) and $\alpha = 0.05$

β	0.50	0.40	0.30	0.20	0.10	0.05
$(z_\alpha + z_{2\beta})^2$	3.842	4.897	6.172	7.849	10.507	12.995

● **Worked example**

Sample size calculation for a study using a parallel design, where two drugs (A and B) are being compared for the treatment of hypertension. The outcome measure of interest is the systolic blood pressure measurement:

Power required (1 – type II error)   0.9 or 90%

Significance level or type I error   0.05 or 5%

Standard deviation of systolic blood pressure measurements   30 mmHg

Smallest clinically important difference to be detected   20 mmHg

Using the formula for comparing the means of two independent samples, the total sample size required is:

$$n = \frac{2 \times 10.507 \times 900}{400} = 96 \text{ in each group}$$

See CAMPBELL and MACHIN (1993) for more worked examples. CLINSTAT, (BLAND, 1991), can perform a number of power calculations.

Appendix B
Choosing the appropriate statistical test

● **Points to consider when choosing a statistical test/method for data analysis**

1. purpose of analysis
2. type of data; assumptions
3. study design: paired data/independent data
4. number of groups

● **Making comparisons**

Categorical data

A. UNPAIRED DATA

　　1. Two groups

　　　　(i) Two outcomes (e.g. dead/alive; yes/no)

　　　　　　χ^2 test

　　　　　　Fisher's exact test

　　　　　　Logistic regression

　　　　　　Log rank test (survival data)

　　　　(ii) More than two outcomes – unordered (e.g. myocardial infarction/pericarditis/pneumonia/oesophagitis)

　　　　　　χ^2 test

　　　　　　Polytomous or multinomial logistic regression

　　　　(iii) More than two outcomes – ordered (e.g. no pain/moderate pain/severe pain)

　　　　　　χ^2 test for trend

　　　　　　Ordered logistic regression

　　2. More than two groups

　　　　(i) Two outcomes

　　　　　　χ^2 test

　　　　　　Logistic regression

　　　　　　Log rank test (survival data)

　　　　(ii) More than two outcomes – groups and outcome unordered

　　　　　　χ^2 test

　　　　　　Polytomous logistic regression

(iii) More than two outcomes – where either the groups or the outcome are ordered
Kruskal–Wallis test
(iv) More than two outcomes – where both the groups and the outcome are ordered
Rank correlation

B. PAIRED DATA
1. Two categories
McNemar's test
Conditional logistic regression
2. More than two categories
(i) Unordered
Stuart–Maxwell test
(ii) Ordered
Wilcoxon matched pairs signed rank test

Quantitative data

A. UNPAIRED DATA
1. Two groups
Independent samples *t*-test
Mann–Whitney *U*-test
Regression/ANCOVA
2. More than two unordered groups
Analysis of variance
Kruskal–Wallis test
Regression/ANCOVA
3. More than two ordered groups
Analysis of variance using linear contrasts
Cuszick's test
Regression/ANCOVA

B. PAIRED DATA
1. Two sets of measurements
Paired *t*-test
Wilcoxon matched pairs signed rank test
2. More than two sets of repeated measurements
Special methods for repeated measurements

● **Assessing relationships**

Strength of associations

A. CATEGORICAL DATA
χ^2 test
Logistic regression methods

B. QUANTITATIVE DATA
Pearson's correlation/rank correlation
Regression

Prediction of outcomes

A. CATEGORICAL DATA
1. Binary
Logistic regression and conditional logistic regression
2. More than two unordered categories
Polytomous logistic regression
3. More than two ordered categories
Ordered logistic regression

B. COUNT DATA AND RATES
Poisson regression

C. SURVIVAL DATA
Cox regression

D. QUANTITATIVE DATA
Linear regression/ANCOVA

● **Confounding and interaction**

Stratification/Mantel–Haenszel methods
Standardization (confounding)
Multiple regression (including logistic, Cox and Poisson regression)

Appendix C
Worked examples for simple significance tests

- **Categorical data**

χ^2-test and z-test for two independent groups

WORKED EXAMPLE

Study in which 50 patients undergoing a new type of surgery, and 50 patients undergoing the standard surgical procedure are asked whether they have experienced severe postsurgical pain:

	New surgery	Standard surgery	Total
Severe pain	5 (10%)	12 (24%)	17
No severe pain	45	38	83
Total	50	50	100

Two different tests can be performed to compare the proportions with severe pain in the two treatment groups: the χ^2-test (commonly used), and the z-test for proportions (which uses the same information necessary for constructing confidence intervals).

χ^2-test

The first step after laying out the contingency table with the observed frequencies and totals, is to calculate the expected frequencies, under the null hypothesis that the proportions with severe pain are the same in the standard and new surgery groups:

	New surgery	Standard surgery	Total
Severe pain	8.5 (17%)	8.5 (17%)	17
No severe pain	41.5	41.5	83
Total	50	50	100

χ^2-statistic is calculated as:

$$\sum \frac{(O-E)^2}{E} = \frac{(5-8.5)^2}{8.5} + \frac{(12-8.5)^2}{8.5} + \frac{(45-41.5)^2}{41.5} + \frac{(38-41.5)^2}{41.5} = 3.472$$

Number of degrees of freedom (df) = 1, i.e. (2 columns − 1) × (2 rows − 1)

P-value = 0.062 (the critical value for $P \leq 0.05$ is 3.84, i.e. the statistic must be ≥ 3.84 for $P \leq 0.05$ with 1 df)

z-test

The z statistic is calculated by dividing the result obtained (here, the difference in proportion with severe pain between the two groups) by its standard error (SE).

Difference in proportions or percentages:

$$0.10 - 0.24 = -0.14 \text{ or } 10\% - 24\% = -14\%$$

SE of the difference between two proportions:

$$SE = \sqrt{\frac{p_1(1 - p_1)}{n_1} + \frac{p_2(1 - p_2)}{n_2}}$$

$$= \sqrt{\frac{0.1 \times 0.9}{50} + \frac{0.24 \times 0.76}{50}} = 0.0738 = 7.38\%$$

z-statistic = $-0.14/0.0738 = -1.897$

P-value = 0.062

95% CI for difference between proportions:
-28% to 0.5% (from 28% less in the new surgery group to 0.5% less in the standard surgery group; CIs cannot be obtained with χ^2-test):

$$95\% \; CI = \text{ difference } \pm \; 1.96 \; SE_{difference}$$

INTERPRETATION

These results suggest the proportion of patients experiencing severe pain is greater with the standard than with the new surgical procedure (24% vs 10%, respectively). However, the results are not conclusive since both the P-value and the 95% confidence interval fail to rule out the possibility that the two treatments are equally effective in preventing severe postsurgical pain.

McNemar's χ^2-test for two paired proportions

WORKED EXAMPLE

Study in which 70 patients suspected of having a particular condition were investigated using two different diagnostic tests:

		Test B		
		Yes	No	Total
	Yes	24	5 (r)	29
Test A	No	9 (s)	32	41
	Total	33	37	70

χ^2-statistic for paired proportions:

$$\chi^2_{\text{paired}} = \frac{(r-s)^2}{r+s} = \frac{(5-9)^2}{5+9} = 1.143$$

where r and s and the numbers of discordant pairs.

Number of degrees of freedom (df) = 1 (2 × 2 table)

P-value > 0.05, since χ^2-statistic <3.84

Difference between paired proportions:

$$(r-s)/n = (5-9)/70 = -0.057 \text{ or } 5.7\%$$

Standard error of difference between paired proportions:

$$\text{SE} = \frac{\sqrt{(r-s)}}{n} = \frac{\sqrt{14}}{70} = \frac{3.742}{70} = 0.053$$

95% CI is calculated as:

$$95\% \text{ CI} = \frac{(r-s)}{n} \pm 1.96 \frac{\sqrt{(r+s)}}{n}$$

In this case, from -0.161 to 0.047.

INTERPRETATION

The difference in proportion with positive diagnosis between the two tests is 0.057 or 5.7%, the proportion of positives being greater for test B. The 95% CI suggests this difference could be as high as 16% higher for test B, or, 4.7% higher for test A. This also indicates the difference observed is not statistically significant ($P > 0.05$).

● **Quantitative data**

t-test for two independent groups

WORKED EXAMPLE

Study in which diastolic blood pressure measurements (DBP) in mmHg are compared in two groups of hypertensive patients with the same baseline levels, who are given two alternative drug treatments:

	Mean	SD	n
Group 1	91 mmHg	5.5	41
Group 2	95 mmHg	5.5	43

Difference in mean DBP = -4 mmHg

SE of difference between two means (equal variance or SD):

$$\text{SE} = \sqrt{(\text{SD}^2/n_1 + \text{SD}^2/n_2)} = 1.20$$

t-statistic = $-4/1.20 = -3.333$

Degrees of freedom (df) = (41 − 2) + (43 − 1) = 82

P-value = 0.0013 (this result is looked up in tables of the t-distribution, with 82 df; the critical value of t for $P \leq 0.05$ is 1.99)

95% CI for difference between means:

$$95\% \text{ CI} = \text{difference} \pm t \times \text{SE}_{\text{difference}}$$

In this case, from −6.39 to −1.61 mmHg.

INTERPRETATION

The difference in mean DBP between the groups compared is statistically significant. The results show the drug administered in group 1 to be more effective in reducing DBP levels. The observed difference of 4 mmHg in favour of group 1, could in fact be greater, 6.39 mmHg, but could also be smaller, 1.61 mmHg.

t-test for paired groups

WORKED EXAMPLE

Study in which the birthweight (in pounds) of a small group of newborns is measured by two different methods:

ID	Method A	Method B	Difference
1	8.9	8.5	−0.4
2	9.0	8.8	−0.2
3	6.7	6.6	−0.1
4	6.3	6.3	0.0
5	7.4	7.5	0.1
6	5.9	6.0	0.1
7	6.5	6.7	0.2
8	8.2	8.4	0.2
9	7.9	8.1	0.2
10	7.5	7.8	0.3

Mean difference in birthweight = 0.04 pounds

SE of mean birthweight difference:

$$SE = \frac{SD}{\sqrt{n}} = \frac{0.217}{3.162} = 0.069$$

t-statistic = 0.04/0.069 = 0.580

Degrees of freedom (df) = (10 − 1) = 9

P-value = 0.574 (this result is looked up in tables of the t-distribution, with 9 df; the critical value of t for $P \leq 0.05$ is 2.26, with 9 df)

95% CI for mean difference:

95% CI = mean difference $\pm$ t $\times$ SE$_{\text{mean difference}}$

In this case, from -0.116 to 0.196 pounds.

INTERPRETATION

The average difference between two weight measurements made by these two methods is 0.04 pounds, method B giving slightly higher measurements on average. The difference between the methods is not statistically significant (which was to be expected given that the two methods are measuring the same 10 babies). The mean difference between the methods could be from 0.196 pounds higher for method B to 0.116 higher for method A. (Note: with small samples the distribution of the differences between paired measurements must have an approximate normal distribution; when this is not the case, non-parametric methods may be preferable to the t-test.)

Appendix D
Worked examples for agreement/reliability of clinical measurements

● **Categorical data**

Kappa **statistic**

WORKED EXAMPLE (SAME AS FOR MCNEMAR'S TEST)
Study in which 70 patients suspected of having a particular condition were investigated using two different diagnostic tests:

		Test B		
		Yes	No	Total
	Yes	24 (13.6)	5	29
Test A	**No**	9	32 (21.6)	41
	Total	33	37	70

Note: numbers in brackets indicate expected frequencies in cells denoting agreement

$$\kappa = 1 - \frac{\text{observed disagreement}}{\text{disagreement expected by chance}}$$

Observed disagreement $= 20.0\%$ $(5/70 + 9/70 = 7.1\% + 12.9\%)$

Disagreement expected by chance $= 1 - (\text{agreement expected by chance})$

$$= 1 - [(13.6 + 21.6)/70] = 1 - 0.503 = 0.497 \text{ or } 49.7\%$$

$$\kappa = 1 - (20.0/49.7) = 0.60$$

INTERPRETATION

For reasons already discussed under κ statistic, the value of κ is difficult to interpret. Nonetheless, the following guide is frequently given in the literature for a rough assessment:

κ	Strength of agreement
<0.01	Poor
0.01–0.20	Slight
0.21–0.40	Fair
0.41–0.60	Moderate
0.61–0.80	Substantial
0.81–1.00	Almost perfect

Note: the P-value associated with a given result for κ does not indicate the strength of agreement, but simply whether the observed agreement, of *whatever* magnitude, is likely to be due to chance.

● **Quantitative data**

Repeatability and reliability

WORKED EXAMPLE (SAME AS FOR PAIRED t-TEST, ASSUMING REPEATED
    MEASUREMENTS MADE USING THE SAME METHOD)

Study in which the birthweight (in pounds) of a small group of newborns is measured twice using the same method:

ID	Method A	Method B	Difference	Squared diff
1	8.9	8.5	−0.4	0.16
2	9.0	8.8	−0.2	0.04
3	6.7	6.6	−0.1	0.01
4	6.3	6.3	0.0	0.00
5	7.4	7.5	0.1	0.01
6	5.9	6.0	0.1	0.01
7	6.5	6.7	0.2	0.04
8	8.2	8.4	0.2	0.04
9	7.9	8.1	0.2	0.04
10	7.5	7.8	0.3	0.09
			Sum	0.44

Mean difference in birthweight = 0.04 pounds

Variance of errors = observed disagreement:

$$\text{Variance of errors} = \frac{\sum(\text{differences})^2}{2n} = \frac{0.44}{20} = 0.022$$

$$\text{SD of errors} = \sqrt{(\text{variance of errors})} = 0.148$$

Reliability of measurements:

$$R = 1 - \frac{\text{observed disagreement}}{\text{chance-expected disagreement}} = 1 - \frac{0.022}{1.02} = 0.98$$

Chance-expected disagreement = variance of all measurements = 1.02

INTERPRETATION

Interpretation of the coefficient of reliability depends on the variance of the measurements in question, which in this case can be considered to be low. Nonetheless, a value for R of 0.98 is considered to represent high reliability. This is the proportion of variability in this set of measurements which is explained by natural variation in birthweight, and consequently, not due to measurement error.

References

Altman D (1991). *Practical Statistics for Medical Research*. Chapman & Hall.

Andersen B (1990). *Methodological Errors in Medical Research*. Blackwell Scientific Publications.

Bland M (1991). *CLINSTAT*. St. George's Hospital Medical School.

Bland M (1995). *An Introduction to Medical Statistics*. Oxford Medical Publications.

Bland M, Altman D (1986). Statistical methods for assessing agreement between two methods of clinical measurement. *The Lancet* i: 307–310.

Campbell M, Machin D (1993). *Medical Statistics. A Common Sense Approach*. Wiley.

Chalmers I, Altman D (eds) (1995). *Systematic Reviews*. BMJ Publishing.

Chatellier G, Zapletal E, Lemaitre D, Menard J, Degoulet P (1996). The number to treat: a clinically useful nomogram in its proper context. *Br Med J* **312**: 426–429, 563.

Clayton D, Hills M (1993). *Statistical Models in Epidemiology*. Oxford University Press.

Dawson-Saunders B, Trapp R (1994). *Basic and Clinical Biostatistics*. Appleton & Lange.

Doll R, Peto R, Wheatley K, Gray R, Sutherland I (1994). Mortality in relation to smoking: 40 years' observations on male British doctors. *Br Med J* **309**: 901–911.

Dunn G, Everitt B (1995). *Clinical Biostatistics: An Introduction to Evidence Based Medicine*. Arnold.

Drummond M (1994). *Economic Analysis Alongside Controlled Trials. An Introduction for Clinical Researchers*. Department of Health.

Fagan TJ (1975). Nomogram from Bayes' theorem. *N Engl J Med* **293**: 257.

Gardner M, Altman D (eds) (1989). *Statistics with Confidence: Confidence Intervals and Statistical Guidelines*. BMJ Publishing.

Gardner S, Winter P, Gardner M (1991). *CIA: Confidence Interval Analysis*. BMJ Publishing.

Gore S, Altman D (eds) (1982). *Statistics in Practice*. BMJ Publishing.

Hamilton L (1997). *Statistics with Stata 5*. Duxbury Press.

ISIS Collaborative Group (1988). Randomized trial of streptokinase, oral aspirin, both, or neither among 17,187 cases of suspected acute myocardial infarction: ISIS-2. *The Lancet* **ii**: 349–359.

Kirkwood B (1988). *Essentials of Medical Statistics*. Blackwell Scientific Publications.

Law M, Cheng R, Hackshaw A, Allaway S, Hale A (1997). Cigarette smoking, sex hormones and bone density in women. *Eur J Epidemiology* **13**: 553–558.

Mann J, Inman W, Thorogood M (1968). Oral contraceptive use in older women and fatal myocardial infarction. *Br Med J* **2**: 193–199.

Matthews J, Altman D, Campbell M, Royston P (1990). Analysis of serial measurements in medical research. *Br Med J* **300**: 230–235.

Pocock S (1983). *Clinical Trials: A Practical Approach*. Wiley.

Roberts M, Alexander F, Anderson T, Forrest A, Hepburn W, Huggins A, Kirkpatrick A, Lamb J, Lutz W, Muir B (1984). The Edinburgh randomised trial of screening for breast cancer: description of method. *Br J Cancer* **50**: 1–6.

Rothman K (1986). *Modern Epidemiology*. Little, Brown & Co.

Sackett D (1979). Bias in analytical research. *J Chron Dis* **32**: 51–63.

Sackett D, Haynes B, Guyatt G, Tugwell P (1991). *Clinical Epidemiology: A Basic Science for Clinical Medicine*. Little, Brown & Co.

Sackett D, Richardson W, Rosenberg W, Haynes B (1997). *Evidence-Based Medicine; How to Practice and Teach EBM*. Churchill Livingstone.

Silfverdal S, Bodin L, Hugosson S, Garpenholt O, Werner B, Esbjorner E, Lindquist B, Olcen P (1997). Protective effect of breastfeeding on invasive haemophilus influenzae infection: a case-control study in Swedish preschool children. *Int J Epidemiol* **26**: 443–450.

Smith G, Song F, Sheldon T (1993). Cholesterol lowering and mortality: the importance of considering initial level of risk. *Br Med J* **306**: 1367–1373.

STATA Corporation (1997). *STATA Statistical Software release 5*. College Station, TX: STATA Corporation.

van Crevel H, Habbema J, Braakman R (1986). Decision analysis of the management of incidental intracranial saccular aneurysms. *Neurology* **36**: 1335–1339.

Wald N (1996). *The Epidemiological Way*. London: Wolfson Institute of Preventative Medicine.

Weinshenker B, Penman M, Bass B, Ebers G, Rice G (1992). A double-blind, randomized crossover trial of pemoline in fatigue associated with multiple sclerosis. *Neurology* **42**: 1468–1471.

Basic statistics series published in the *Canadian Medical Association Journal* (Guyatt G, Jaeschke R, Heddle N, Cook D, Shannon H, Walter S):

1   Hypothesis testing. *CMAJ* 1995, **151(1)**: 27–32.

2   Interpreting study intervals: confidence intervals. *CMAJ* 1995, **152(2)**: 169–173.

3   Assessing the effects of treatment: measures of association. *CMAJ* 1995, **152(3)**: 351–357.

4   Correlation and regression. *CMAJ* 1995, **152(4)**: 497–504.

'Users' Guides to the Medical Literature' published in the *Journal of the American Medical Association* (Evidence-Based Medicine Working Group):

I   How to get started. *JAMA* 1993, **270(17)**: 2093–2095.

II   How to use an article about therapy and prevention.

     A. Are the results of the study valid? *JAMA* 1993, **270(21)**: 2598–2601.

II   How to use an article about therapy and prevention.

     B. What are the results and will they help me in caring for my patients? *JAMA* 1994, **271(1)**: 59–63.

III How to use an article about a diagnostic test.

     A. Are the results of the study valid? *JAMA* 1994, **271(5)**: 389–391.

III How to use an article about a diagnostic test.

     B. What are the results and will they help me in caring for my patients? *JAMA* 1994, **271(9)**: 703–707.

IV   How to use an article about harm. *JAMA* 1994, **271(20)**: 1615–1619.

V   How to use an article about prognosis. *JAMA* 1994, **272(3)**: 234–237.

VI   How to use an overview. *JAMA* 1994, **272(17)**: 1367–1371.

VII How to use a clinical decision analysis.

     A. Are the results of the study valid? *JAMA* 1995, **273(16)**: 1292–1295.

VII How to use a clinical decision analysis.

     B. What are the results and will they help me in caring for my patients? *JAMA* 1995, **273(20)**: 1610–1613.

VIII How to use clinical practice guidelines.

     A. Are the recommendations valid? *JAMA* 1995, **274(7)**: 570–574.

IX   A method for grading health care recommendations. *JAMA* 1995; **274**: 1800–1804.

XII How to use articles about health-related quality of life. *JAMA* 1997; **277**: 1232–1237.

XIII Drummond M, Richardson W, O'Brien B, Levine M, Heyland D. How to use an economic analysis.

A. Are the results valid? *JAMA* 1997, **277(19)**: 1552–1557.

XIII O'Brien B, Heyland D, Richardson W, Levine M, Drummond M. How to use an economic analysis.

B. What are the results and will they help me in caring for my patients? *JAMA* 1997, **277(22)**: 1802–1806.

Other medical statistics dictionaries

Armitage P, Colton T (eds) (1998). *Encyclopedia of Biostatistics*, (six volumes). John Wiley.

Everitt B (1995). *Dictionary of Statistics in the Medical Sciences*. Cambridge University Press.

Last J (1995). *A Dictionary of Epidemiology*. Oxford University Press.

Index